RADIOLOGICAL DIAGNOSIS
OF DIGESTIVE TRACT DISORDERS
IN THE NEWBORN

Radiological Diagnosis
of Digestive

A GUIDE TO RADIOLOGISTS

B. J. Cremin
D.(OBST.)R.C.O.G., M.C.R.A., F.F.R.

Principal Specialist in
Radiology, Red Cross
War Memorial
Children's Hospital,
Cape Town, South Africa

LONDON

Tract Disorders
in the Newborn

URGEONS AND PAEDIATRICIANS

S. Cywes
M.MED.(Surg.)

*ssociate Professor
nd Principal Surgeon,
ed Cross War
Memorial Children's
ospital, Cape Town,
outh Africa*

J. H. Louw
Ch.M., F.R.C.S.

*Professor of Surgery,
University of Cape Town,
and Groote Schuur and
Red Cross War
Memorial Children's
Hospitals, Cape Town,
South Africa*

BUTTERWORTHS

ENGLAND: BUTTERWORTH & CO. (PUBLISHERS) LTD.
LONDON: 88 Kingsway, WC2B 6AB

AUSTRALIA: BUTTERWORTHS PTY. LTD.
SYDNEY: 586 Pacific Highway, 2067
MELBOURNE: 343 Little Collins Street, 3000
BRISBANE: 240 Queen Street, 4000

CANADA: BUTTERWORTH & CO. (CANADA) LTD.
TORONTO: 14 Curity Avenue, 374

NEW ZEALAND: BUTTERWORTHS OF NEW ZEALAND LTD
WELLINGTON: 26–28 Waring Taylor Street, 1

SOUTH AFRICA: BUTTERWORTH & CO. (SOUTH AFRICA) (PTY) LTD.
DURBAN: 152–154 Gale Street

Suggested U.D.C. Number: 616-037·75 : 61613-053·31

ISBN 0 407 38375 1

Made and printed in Great Britain by
William Clowes & Sons, Limited, London, Beccles and Colchester

Preface

Disorders of the digestive tract in the newborn are a major cause of infant mortality. Most of the lesions are congenital in origin and are responsible for a life-threatening situation requiring prompt surgical correction. Early and accurate diagnosis is therefore of paramount importance and this depends largely on clinical observations and the correct interpretation of radiographs. The clinical and radiographic data must be complementary to each other. The radiologist must be aware of the clinical possibilities while the clinician should be able to interpret the radiological findings.

In this book we have attempted to outline the essential clinical and radiological features in such a way that they can be used as a guide by both radiologists and clinicians. The text has been deliberately condensed for the sake of brevity and particular emphasis has been placed on illustrated radiographs. In each section our techniques for the radiological examination of the sick infant are described. These methods are intended to act as a guide for those who have not had the opportunity of developing their own skills, and should not be regarded as rigid rules. Nevertheless, it is our firm belief that the radiologist must have the necessary equipment for adequate image intensification fluoroscopy. This not only reduces the amount of radiation exposure but often enables the correct diagnosis to be made at the time of the examination. We realize that the methods of examination advised may only be possible in the more sophisticated departments of large paediatric hospitals. We make no excuse for this because we believe that the sick infant deserves nothing but the best that can be offered.

All the radiographs are of the newborn infant (up to four weeks of age) with the exceptions of *Figures 1.5* (six months), *1.9* (ten months),

3.9 (one year), and *5.8* (three years). These four examples were chosen to illustrate the radiological features of particular maladies seen in young infants. Many of the diagnostic points have been culled from the American, British, and Continental radiological journals of the past ten years. Similarly, much of the clinical information comes from the many recent standard textbooks and journals on paediatric surgery. We have, however, reduced our bibliography to a minimum and limited it to the important or recent publications from which many of the references used by us may be obtained. We thank all the authors concerned.

We wish to acknowledge the source of the following illustrations: Dr. P. Franklyn of Bradford, Dr. H. Kaufmann of Philadelphia, Dr. J. Moir and the *Journal of the Canadian Association of Radiologists* for *Figures 1.9, 3.7,* and *3.8a* and *b* respectively. We thank them for the loan of these films and permission to publish them.

We also wish to thank the undermentioned journals for permission to re-publish from our own articles the following illustrations:

Figure 2.15: American Journal of Roentgenology
Figure 3.6: Radiology
Figure 4.11: Journal of Pediatric Surgery
Figures 5.10, 5.12: South African Medical Journal
Figure 6.1: Annales de Radiologie
Figures 6.6a and b, 6.9, 6.12: Surgery
Figures 6.6c, 6.10, 6.11, 6.14a and b, 6.15 and 6.16: Clinical Radiology

We would like to thank everyone who assisted in the preparation of this book. Special mention must be made of the Red Cross Hospital medical staff (particularly the radiographers and radiologists) and photographic staff, Mrs. D. Ladegaard and Mrs. U. Barrett; also Mr. P. Wheeler and Mrs. O. Enslin of the Department of Surgery, Illustration Section, and those who patiently typed and re-typed the manuscript, foremost amongst whom have been Miss D. Wilson and Miss L. Malan.

B.J.C.
S.C.
J.H.L.

Contents

1

Oesophageal Lesions and Diaphragmatic Hernias

OESOPHAGEAL ATRESIA AND TRACHEO-OESOPHAGEAL FISTULAE

Atresia is the most common and most important congenital abnormality of the oesophagus. The incidence is generally quoted as 1 case in 3,000 live births, but the anomaly is probably more common because some cases may succumb to pneumonia without a correct diagnosis having been made.

The malformation occurs in the proximal oesophagus about 1–3 cm below the superior constrictor muscle, i.e., at approximately the level of the second dorsal vertebra (9–12 cm from the upper gum margin). In 90% of patients it is associated with a tracheo-oesophageal fistula, which usually communicates with the lower oesophageal segment, but may communicate with the upper, and even with both. Distal fistulae usually communicate with the trachea 0·5–1 cm above the carina, but may enter the trachea up to 2 cm more proximally, or as far distally as the first centimetre of either bronchus. Very rarely the fistula exists without atresia (H-fistula). The anatomical variations have been classified in many ways and the following is the classification currently used (*Figure 1.1a–e*).

(a) *Atresia without fistula (10%):* the upper segment tends to be longer than those associated with a fistula and the lower segment is usually short, with a long gap between the segments.

(b) *Atresia with fistula between proximal segment and trachea:* this is excessively rare, accounting for 0·5–1% of cases reported in various large series.

(c) *Atresia with fistula between distal segment and trachea:* this is the common variety, accounting for almost 90% of cases. There are marked variations between the distance of the proximal and distal segments, the average distance being 1–2 cm. Occasionally the segments overlap, with some continuity of the oesophageal walls. Very rarely the lumen of the fistula is so minute that air does not pass through it.

1

(d) *Atresia with fistulae between both proximal and distal segments of the trachea:* this is also extremely rare, occurring in less than 1% of cases.

(e) *Fistula without atresia (H-fistula):* this variety, which is difficult to diagnose, accounts for 1–3% of cases. The fistula is usually a

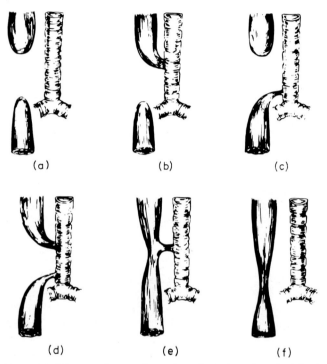

(a)   (b)   (c)

(d)   (e)   (f)

Figure 1.1. Diagram of types of oesophageal atresia and tracheal fistula

single narrow slit, frequently situated at a relatively high level (region of the clavicle or higher) but also occurring at midtrachea or lower levels. Very rarely there may be a double H-fistula.

(f) Congenital oesophageal stenosis (*Figure 1.1 f—see* p. 9).

Clinical presentation and diagnosis

Maternal hydramnios

Any anomaly which prevents the foetus from ingesting or absorbing amniotic fluid will enhance the development of hydramnios. All atresias of the alimentary tract are, therefore, associated with an increased incidence of hydramnios. This applies particularly to oesophageal atresia without fistula, where the incidence may be as high as 85%; however, when a fistula communicates with the distal segment the incidence drops to 30%. In view of these figures, the presence of hydramnios should always raise the possibility of oesophageal atresia in the infant and prompt the passage of a nasogastric tube for diagnostic purposes.

Prematurity

About 30% of infants with oesophageal atresia are premature. Although this is not of diagnostic significance, it is of great importance as far as management and prognosis are concerned.

Associated congenital anomalies

Additional congenital abnormalities are present in more than 50% of infants with oesophageal atresia; approximately half of them are incompatible with life or at best will permit only a limited life expectancy unless correctable by surgery. The systems most frequently involved are the following:

Cardiovascular	25%
Rectum and anus	10%
Rest of gastro-intestinal tract	10%
Genito-urinary	5%

Multiple anomalies are often present and are significant major disabilities in about 10% of cases, a relatively common combination being oesophageal atresia, duodenal atresia, and anorectal agenesis. The presence of any of the above anomalies should prompt investigation to determine the presence or absence of oesophageal atresia.

Symptoms and signs

The following should alert the clinician:

(a) *A moist neonate* with a frothing, wet mouth often blowing bubbles. The baby is unable to swallow and therefore an excessive amount of mucus and saliva flow from the mouth. As the saliva accumulates the baby may cough, choke, or regurgitate and become dyspnoeic and cyanotic. Symptoms become more evident during attempts at feeding and if these are continued the infant may die from aspiration of the feed or pneumonia.

(b) *Persistent pneumonitis:* a significant number of these infants present with pulmonary problems due to pneumonitis. This may be diffuse or confined to the upper lobes, especially the right upper lobe which is particularly prone to atelectasis and infection.

3

When oesophageal atresia is suspected, the diagnosis should be confirmed by passing a relatively thick (French gauge 10 or 12) rubber catheter down the nose into the oesophagus. If the catheter meets an obstruction at 9 to 12 cm from the anterior nares, the diagnosis is established. However, the tube may become curled up in the oesophagus and the impression may be gained that it has entered the stomach (*Figure 1.2*). Moreover, the aspiration of large quantities of secretion from the upper pouch may support this

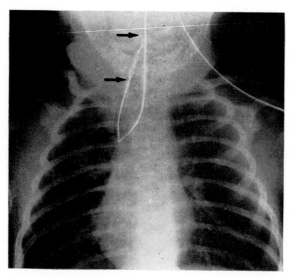

Figure 1.2. Radio-opaque catheter curled up in proximal oesophageal pouch

impression, particularly if bile-stained material, which has been regurgitated from the stomach via the fistula, is present. (Still greater confusion may arise if the tube is inadvertently introduced into the trachea and passed through the fistula into the distal segment of the oesophagus and stomach.) If an obstruction is met the catheter should be replaced by a double lumen Replogle tube which is attached to constant low-pressure suction to keep the upper blind pouch empty and the infant taken for radiological confirmation of the diagnosis.

Radiological diagnosis

Plain films of chest and abdomen

If the condition has not been suspected on clinical grounds and the infant is referred for radiological examination, the plain films of the chest and abdomen may provide the following information:

(1) *Abnormal gas shadows:* an airless abdomen should suggest an oesophageal atresia without a fistula or the associated rarities of a proximal fistula or blocked distal fistula. When air is present, then the common atresia with a distal fistula may be suspected. The intestinal air is frequently excessive in amount but if there is a lack of air and fluid levels are present, additional atresias should also be suspected.

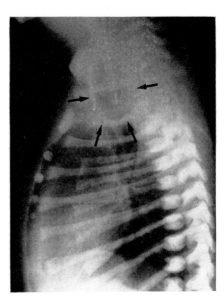

Figure 1.3. Radio-opaque catheter in proximal oesophageal pouch; the pouch is outlined with air injected just prior to the exposure

(2) Presence of *pneumonitis*, especially in the right upper lobe.
(3) *Cardiac anomalies.*
(4) *Skeletal anomalies.*

Plain films with catheter in position
The AP and lateral chest films are of value in checking the site of the catheter. A Replogle tube is easily identified because of its width and the presence of the longitudinal radio-opaque stripe, and it is best seen on the lateral chest films. A moment before the film is exposed 25–50 ml of air should be injected down the tube to outline the upper pharyngeal pouch (*Figure 1.3*).

It is not necessary to use contrast material, but if used judiciously,

5

no harm should result. The technique employed is more important than the type of contrast medium. Only 1 ml of contrast should be drawn into the syringe and only a drop injected into the blind pouch under fluoroscopic control, with the baby in the lateral position (*Figure 1.4*). When the atresia has been identified and a spot film taken, the contrast material must be aspirated from the pouch.

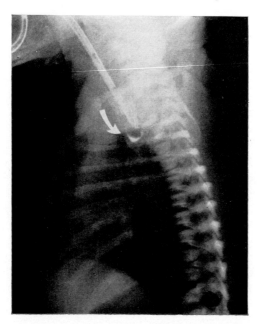

Figure 1.4. Contrast injection demonstrating an oesophageal atresia; we do not advise this method but, if performed, one drop only should be injected

If this technique is employed there is no reason why barium should not be used, because even if the drop that has been injected is regurgitated into the lungs, it is rapidly coughed up without adverse effects. Some radiologists prefer to use Dionosil or a water soluble contrast material such as Gastrografin, but the latter is hypertonic and may cause irritation if aspirated.

Identification of the fistula

This is necessary in the H-fistula which usually presents later in infancy with recurrent attacks of pneumonia. The opening of the fistula is a narrow, longitudinal slit and difficult to visualize by endoscopy. However, blue dye instilled into the oesophagus may pass through the fistula into the trachea where it can be seen emerging on bronchoscopy.

Radiographic identification is more satisfactory and best carried out with the infant placed in the prone position on the elevated foot-rest of an erect screening table. A nasogastric tube is passed into the stomach and small amounts of contrast material injected at intervals whilst the catheter is slowly withdrawn (*Figure 1.5*). A water soluble contrast medium may be used but the injection of carefully controlled amounts of dilute barium is a safe method to demonstrate a small fistula. The fistula usually shows only momentarily and the small amount of contrast material is rapidly coughed up. The whole oesophagus should be examined, but particular attention must be paid to the upper third to detect the passage of the contrast medium

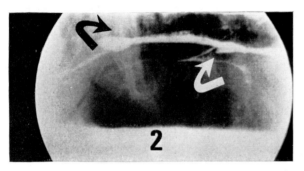

Figure 1.5. 'H' type oesophageal fistula; 70 mm camera study, infant prone and the catheter withdrawn to the level of the clavicles (black arrow), fistula into trachea is demonstrated (white arrow)

into the bronchial tree. This should be differentiated from overflow with nasopharyngeal aspiration into the lungs. Image intensification is essential and the use of a videotape allows for later playback and study. Alternatively, cineradiography at fast speeds of 32 to 48 frames per second may be used, but this is less convenient and also increases the radiation exposure.

With care it is usually possible to make an accurate anatomical diagnosis in patients with oesophageal atresias and tracheo-oesophageal fistulae. The findings may be summarized as follows:

(1) *Atresia without fistula:* a blind pouch in the neck and an airless abdomen (*Figure 1.6*).

(2) *Atresia with fistula between proximal segment and trachea:* findings similar to those in (1), but severe pneumonitis is more likely, and the fistula may be demonstrated if contrast medium is used.

7

(3) *Atresia with fistula between distal segment and trachea:* a blind proximal pouch in the neck with gas in the intestines. In the very rare cases where the lumen of the fistula is excessively minute, the abdomen may be airless.

(4) *Atresia with fistulae between proximal and distal segments:* the

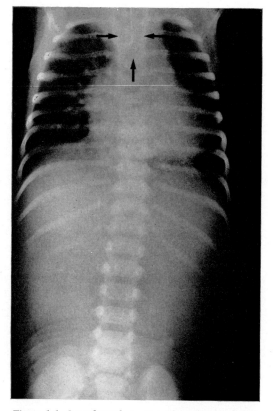

Figure 1.6. Oesophageal atresia without fistula; there is a gasless abdomen and a catheter is present in the upper oesophageal pouch (arrows)

features are similar to those of (3), but severe pneumonitis is more likely and the upper fistula may show up if contrast medium is used.

(5) *H-fistula:* severe pulmonary changes are usually present due to recurrent pneumonitis. The fistula can be visualized by a prone contrast examination with adequate fluoroscopy.

Post-operative radiological examination

Chest

Post-operative films are necessary to follow the course of the aspiration pneumonitis which is frequently present. This usually resolves but residual atelectasis may persist.

Oesophagus

(1) *Integrity of the anastomosis:* a Gastrografin swallow examination should be done before feeding is commenced, and in every case where a leak is suspected. When the anomaly has been corrected by an extra-pleural approach, the first evidence of leakage is likely to be the development of a small pleural effusion. On the other hand, when a transpleural approach has been used a leak is likely to cause a major effusion and/or pneumothorax.

(2) *Recurrence of fistula:* re-establishment of the tracheo-oesophageal communication usually follows a small leak with resultant infection. It leads to respiratory distress on feeding and recurrent pneumonitis which can be assessed on plain films of the chest. The fistula may also be demonstrated with adequate fluoroscopy.

(3) *Stricture:* in the early post-operative period some degree of narrowing at the anastomotic site is often seen on barium swallow examination, and is usually of no significance. If, however, the radiographic narrowing persists and there are feeding problems, a stricture should be suspected. Mild strictures often cause no problems but in later childhood impaction of foreign bodies may lead to acute dysphagia.

(4) *Condition of the lower segment:* following the repair of oesophageal atresia the lower oesophagus often exhibits for some months, abnormal, sluggish, 'yo-yo' movements. In addition, oesophageal reflux with small hiatus hernias is not infrequent and requires follow-up.

OESOPHAGEAL STENOSIS

The commonest cause of oesophageal stricture in infancy is hiatus hernia with reflux peptic oesophagitis, and although it usually occurs in later infancy, it has been reported in the newborn. These strictures affect the lower oesophagus but may extend as far as the mid-oesophagus and even the upper thoracic oesophagus (p. 24).

Congenital stenosis of the oesophagus is extremely rare but has been reported on a number of occasions and is, in fact, regarded as a variant of oesophageal atresia (*Figure 1.1f*) comparable to intestinal stenosis. It usually occurs at the junction of middle and lower thirds of the oesophagus and is seldom severe enough to cause dysphagia at birth. However, superadded inflammatory oedema may lead to complete obstruction with regurgitation of feeds and aspiration pneumonia within a relatively short period.

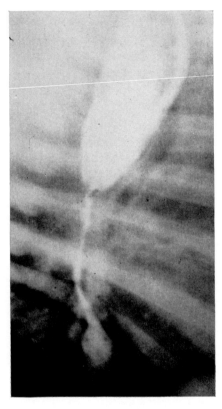

Figure 1.7. Congenital oeso-phageal stenosis; a further study after dilatation showed no evidence of reflux or hernia

The diagnosis can be made on a barium swallow which shows a smooth, abrupt obstruction (*Figure 1.7*). Oesophagoscopy is usually unrewarding because of the inflammatory oedema.

MEDIASTINAL DUPLICATIONS OF FOREGUT ORIGIN

The mediastinum is one of the common sites for duplications of the alimentary canal. Usually they occur as rounded cysts of varying

size in the posterior mediastinum, closely associated with the oesophagus. They have the external appearance of bowel with muscular
walls and are lined by intestinal, gastric, and even ciliated epithelium—hence the alternative designations, enteric, enterogenous, or
gastrogenous cysts. Unlike similar duplication cysts of the bowel,
they are easily separated from the oesophagus and ordinarily do not
communicate with the lumen of the oesophagus. Consequently,
being lined by secretory epithelium, they tend to fill with fluid and
enlarge rapidly enough to cause symptoms in infancy and early

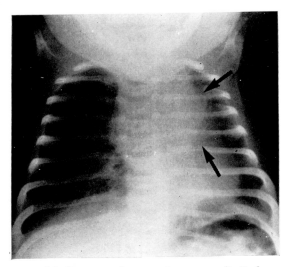

*Figure 1.8. Chest x-ray demonstrating upper mediastinal mass
due to a foregut duplication cyst*

childhood. A rare variant, lined by ciliated epithelium and containing cartilage in its wall, is closely associated with the oesophagus;
often intramural, it expands very slowly and rarely causes symptoms
in the neonate.

Sometimes the duplications are tubular in shape and occasionally
these may penetrate through the diaphragm to end blindly in the
abdomen or to connect with the duodenum or jejunum so that air
or barium may enter the mediastinal portion.

Cervical and upper dorsal vertebral anomalies are often associated
with these mediastinal duplications, for instance, anterior or posterior spina bifida and hemivertebrae. Occasionally the cephalic end
of the duplication is attached to the spine and it may even open into

11

the spinal canal. Very rarely there may be an intestinal fistula pene-trating through a dorsal vertebral defect. All these anomalies are readily explained on a basis of the split notochord syndrome. However, the mediastinal duplications of foregut origin may also be associated with duplications of the midgut, which owe their existence to a different mechanism, and to other intrathoracic malformations such as agenesis of a lung and oesophageal atresia. The rare intramural type of oesophageal duplication is not associated with vertebral anomalies and is probably of bronchogenic origin.

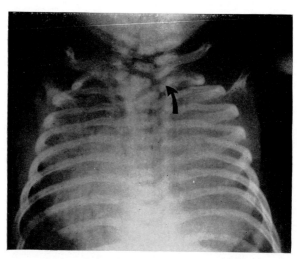

Figure 1.9. Chest x-ray demonstrating a neuroenteric cyst, note the hemivertebrae (arrow) in upper thoracic spine (courtesy of Dr. P. Franklyn, Bradford)

Clinical presentation

Respiratory distress is the principal symptom in the neonate and in Rickham's series more than half the cases presented within the first week of life. Physical signs indicating the presence of a posterior mediastinal mass may be present but, as in all cases of respiratory distress in the newborn, urgent radiological examination is essential to establish the diagnosis.

Radiological diagnosis

Plain AP, lateral, and oblique x-rays of the chest will reveal the presence of a mediastinal mass and its relation to the trachea (*Figure*

1.8). The vertebrae should be carefully scrutinized for abnormalities which are frequently present (*Figure 1.9*). In the rare tubular duplications which communicate with the bowel, a gas shadow may be seen in the mediastinum. A barium swallow is necessary to demonstrate the intimate relationship to the oesophagus (*Figure 1.10a and*

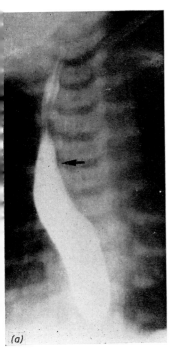 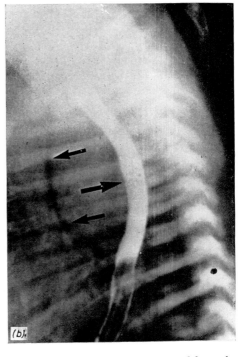

Figure 1.10a. Oesophagus pushed to right by foregut duplication cyst (same case as Figure 1.8)

Figure 1.10b. The trachea is compressed forwards; the main symptom in this two week old infant was stridor, made worse by feeding

b), and to differentiate the mass from other mediastinal masses such as neurogenic tumours and anterior meningocoeles. In the rare variety of mediastinal duplication which communicates with the duodenum or jejunum, barium may enter the structure and show up in the mediastinum. Bronchography is seldom helpful in distinguishing oesophageal duplications from bronchogenic cysts, and it may be impossible to differentiate the intramural type of duplication.

CONGENITAL OESOPHAGEAL DIVERTICULA

The classical pharyngeal pouch of adults is extremely uncommon in infants; the few reported cases have manifested themselves in the newborn period. The symptoms are similar to those of oesophageal atresia and the diagnosis may be missed even on barium swallow

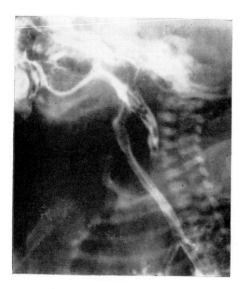

Figure 1.11. Pseudodiverticulum (false passage created by oesophageal catheterization) with free reflux into trachea (the infant arrived at the hospital with these x-rays)

because the contrast material tends to enter the pouch. The alert radiologist should bear this in mind whenever the findings are not typical of atresia and request endoscopy for confirmation of the diagnosis. The same applies to the even more rare diverticula associated with tracheo-oesophageal fistula or oesophageal stenosis.

True diverticula of the body of the oesophagus are probably the rarest of all oesophageal anomalies. Most of the reported cases have occurred in the cervical oesophagus and presented later in life with recurrent respiratory infections or progressive dysphagia. The diagnosis can be made on barium swallow, but endoscopy is necessary to differentiate these lesions from iatrogenic lesions produced by the forceful passage of catheters for the purpose of oesophageal aspiration or feeding (*Figure 1.11*).

VASCULAR RINGS

Anomalous development of the aortic arch and its large branches is only significant when the abnormal vessels compress the trachea and/

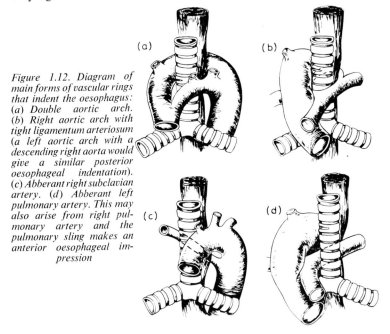

Figure 1.12. Diagram of main forms of vascular rings that indent the oesophagus: (a) Double aortic arch. (b) Right aortic arch with tight ligamentum arteriosum (a left aortic arch with a descending right aorta would give a similar posterior oesophageal indentation). (c) Abberant right subclavian artery. (d) Abberant left pulmonary artery. This may also arise from right pulmonary artery and the pulmonary sling makes an anterior oesophageal impression

or oesophagus; sometimes there are associated congenital heart lesions.

The symptoms are inspiratory stridor, dyspnoea and cyanosis, dysphagia or vomiting, and recurrent chest infections. The infants usually present in the first six months of life and characteristically the dyspnoea and stridor are increased by feeding, when distension of the oesophagus aggravates the compression. Characteristically too, these infants retract their heads during attacks of stridor in an effort to relieve the obstructed airway. All infants presenting with the above symptoms should have a barium swallow to detect the presence of abnormal vessels indenting the oesophagus. This is best seen in the oblique and lateral positions.

The important vascular abnormalities which may occur are illustrated in *Figure 1.12* and include the following:

(a) *Double aortic arch* is the most common anomaly. The double aorta forms a complete vascular ring around the oesophagus and trachea. There is considerable variation in the size of each arch, but the right or posterior component of the ring is usually the larger and causes compression of both trachea and oesophagus. The barium swallow will show a considerable posterior indentation of the oesophagus and there may be a localized anterior indentation at a slightly higher level (*Figure 1.13a*). However, the trachea takes

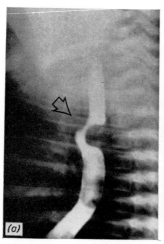 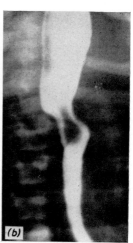

Figure 1.13a. Marked posterior indentation of the oesophagus with compression of trachea anteriorly (arrowhead)

Figure 1.13b. Slight lateral compression of oesophagus

most of the anterior compression and consequently anterior oesophageal indentation may not be seen. Lateral indentations may be seen on the AP view and are likewise slight (*Figure 1.13b*).

(b) *Right aortic arch with a tight ligamentum arteriosum* is similar to a double arch. The trachea is compressed on its right border by the right aortic arch and anteriorly by the pulmonary artery. The ring is completed by a taut ligamentum arteriosum or patent ductus which runs posteriorly from the left pulmonary artery behind the oesophagus to the descending arch of the aorta. The barium swallow will show this as a posterior indentation of the upper oesophagus.

(c) *Aberrant right subclavian artery* does not usually produce symptoms in childhood because the trachea is not compressed. The right subclavian artery arises from the aorta distal to the left subclavian artery and passes up behind the oesophagus to the right side. In doing so it produces an oblique, posterior groove in the oesophagus just above the aortic arch, and this may be responsible for the dysphagia lusoria of adult life. The barium swallow will reveal an oblique indentation of the oesophagus on the AP film.

(d) *Aberrant left pulmonary artery* is rare but occurs when the left pulmonary artery arises to the right of the normal site. In its passage from the main pulmonary trunk to the left lung, it passes between the trachea and oesophagus and may cause compression. This will be seen as an anterior impression of the oesophagus on the barium swallow.

(e) *Other varieties* are anomalies of the origin of the innominate and left carotid arteries. These vessels may arise nearer the midline than normal and compress the trachea anteriorly. They do not compress the oesophagus and therefore no indentation of the oesophagus is seen on barium swallow. Another distinguishing feature is the lack of association between any attacks of stridor and feeding routines.

PHARYNGO-OESOPHAGEAL INCOORDINATION

Functional obstruction at the level of the cricopharyngeus is not common. In this region the lower horizontal fibres of the inferior constrictor muscle blend with the upper circular fibres of the oesophagus. An incomplete relaxation of this area causes liquids to overdistend the pharynx so that retropulsion into the nasopharynx or overflow into the larynx occurs. This is usually an inconstant and transitory phenomenon but may be severe enough to cause grave pulmonary complications. When it occurs, it must be differentiated from a high oesophageal fistula by studying adequate videotape playbacks or cineradiographic recordings taken during swallowing.

ACHALASIA OF THE OESOPHAGUS

Achalasia of the oesophagus, sometimes erroneously referred to as cardiospasm, is extremely uncommon in infants. The condition is due to deficiency of the ganglion cells of Auerbach's plexus, the cause of which is still uncertain. It is characterized by feeble, incoordinate peristalsis in the body of the oesophagus and failure of relaxation of the cardio-oesophageal sphincter. This results in dysphagia, regurgitation, and aspiration pneumonitis.

Barium swallow reveals dilatation of the oesophagus with a smooth

17

tapering at the gastro-oesophageal junction. The feeble, incoordinate peristaltic waves are evident on fluoroscopy and cineradiography. The radiographic appearance must be differentiated from prolonged vestibular spasm (cardiospasm) occasionally encountered in infants. Provided the infant's deglutition reflex is effective, spasm will cause only transient hold-up of the barium. Ineffective propulsive waves with hold-up of barium in the lower oesophagus may also occur in marasmic infants and this, too, must be differentiated from achalasia.

CHALASIA, OESOPHAGEAL REFLUX, AND HIATUS HERNIA

The oesophagus of the normal infant is a muscular tube about 12 cm in length. The upper one-third contains striated muscle and at the junction of this muscle with smooth muscle below, there is a barely discernible constriction of the lumen. This is situated at the level of the tracheal bifurcation. The most distal portion of the oesophagus, the vestibule, lies immediately above, within, and immediately below the oesophageal hiatus of the diaphragm. On spot films it is difficult to correlate the position of the vestibule with the level of the diaphragm, but on fluoroscopy a constricted vestibular area is frequently seen above the diaphragm.

Chalasia

Chalasia is an unfortunate term which should be abolished. It is the name given to a condition encountered in newborn infants and characterized by an apparent relaxation of the cardio-oesophageal sphincter with free reflux of gastric content into the oesophagus. Although a patulous and widely open cardia with reflux may occur in lesions of the central nervous system, we do not accept the concept of chalasia as a distinct entity.

Oesophageal reflux

The mechanisms responsible for the prevention of reflux are not completely understood, but it would appear that the principal factor is the muscular throttle of the vestibular cuff which is assisted by folds of mucosa that act as an inner mucosal choke (*Figure 1.14b*) and by the diaphragmatic crus which acts as an external pinch-cock. Normally the vestibule is closed resulting in a zone of increased intraluminal pressure immediately above the cardia. The factors responsible for the opening of the vestibule are not fully understood, but a number of mechanisms appear to be involved. These may be elucidated by careful radiological examination. In small infants fluoro-

18

scopy and spot films alone are inadequate for the purpose and must be supplemented by playback videotapes that are best obtained from a high quality, pulsed image intensifier. A 70 mm camera with exposures varying from 1 to 6 per second gives good results. When the films are taken at a rate of 1 or 2 per second there is sufficient

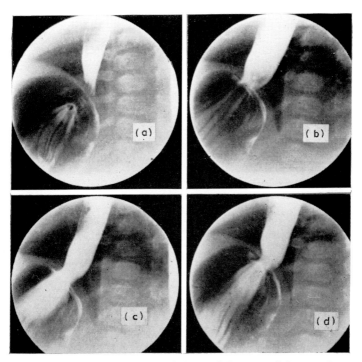

Figure 1.14. The normal function of the vestibular area of the oesophagus shown in sequence by a 70 mm camera study: (a) Vestibule totally closed. (b) Commencement of supradiaphragmatic opening. (c) Vestibule totally open. (d) Commencement of diaphragmatic closure

time between flashes to visualize the oesophagus well enough to obtain an exact image of the film to be taken.

Radiological examination of the infant's oesophagus is carried out with the infant in the horizontal position. Normally a 50% barium suspension is given from a feeding bottle, but in infants who have difficulty in sucking a nasal feeding tube may be used, while in older infants spoon feeding may be necessary. If the infant has been re-ferred for the investigation of unexplained vomiting, the initial swallow is given with the baby in the supine position. A quick glimpse

19

of the oesophagus will suffice to exclude gross lesions, and then the infant should be turned into the prone position for examination of the pylorus and duodenum before too much barium has been given. Careful attention should be paid to the pyloroduodenal area because oesophageal reflux is not uncommon in infants with lesions at these sites. Thereafter the oesophagus is examined in greater detail by giving more barium and keeping the infant in the same prone position with the left side elevated. This position provides an excellent view of the lower oesophagus and vestibule through the gastric air bubble (*Figure 1.14a*). The entrance of the oesophagus into the

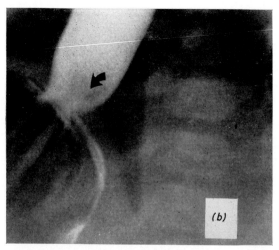

Figure 1.14b. An enlargement showing the mucosal choke (arrow) in action while the vestibule is still closed

stomach has the appearance of an anal canal, and the movements of the vestibule can be clearly seen as it opens and shuts to let barium through.

The act of deglutition starts a propulsive peristaltic wave which passes down the oesophagus and propels the swallowed bolus into the lower oesophagus. If this wave is adequate and the bolus of good size, the vestibule will open when the wave reaches it. The presence of a good bolus seems to be important. Indeed, the vestibule will also open quite normally if barium is injected via a nasal tube into the lower oesophagus. On the other hand, peristaltic waves *per se* do not always empty the oesophagus completely and barium may be held up by independent contractions of the vestibule. These contractions, which may be related to the pinch-cock action of the diaphragmatic crus, are usually intermittent and followed by periods of relaxation which allow a series of squirts of barium into the stomach. Sometimes, however, the vestibule fails to relax at the end of a swallow with retention of a small amount of barium above the cardia. Indeed, occasionally it remains closed despite apparently forceful waves of contraction which may even be seen to bounce back (*Figure 1.15*). Another, and perhaps more important, mechanism is responsible for relaxation of the vestibule. This is the so-called deglutition reflex

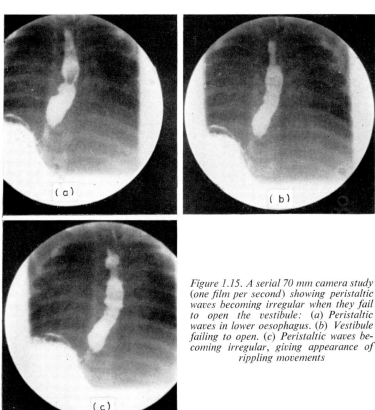

Figure 1.15. A serial 70 mm camera study (one film per second) showing peristaltic waves becoming irregular when they fail to open the vestibule: (a) Peristaltic waves in lower oesophagus. (b) Vestibule failing to open. (c) Peristaltic waves becoming irregular, giving appearance of rippling movements

which is mediated via pharyngeal, vagal, and sympathetic nerves, and is independent of oesophageal peristalsis and even of oesophageal muscular continuity (Chrispin, 1969). The response of the vestibule is initiated by the act of swallowing and follows very shortly after the act and before peristaltic waves reach the lower oesophagus. It may be demonstrated by getting the infant to suck an empty teat

21

which stimulates the act of swallowing and this is a useful manoeuvre in cases where the vestibule remains firmly closed.

In contrast to the cases in whom the vestibule remains closed, there are those where it opens widely and permits free reflux of barium from the stomach into the oesophagus. Fortunately, the oesophagus can hold a considerable amount of regurgitated material and if the reflux is intermittent, subsequent oesophageal contractions may empty the organ before there is spill-over into the pharynx.

Some degree of oesophageal reflux is common in early infancy and no doubt related to the infant's long recumbency in a supine position, the small capacity of the stomach, and the considerable differences between intra-abdominal and intra-thoracic pressure during crying. Moreover, the pinch-cock action of the diaphragmatic crus is not completely effective in the first few months of life. The intermittent reflux of small amounts of gastric contents should, therefore, not be considered abnormal in early infancy.

In infants with significant reflux there is a continuous backflow from the stomach and the oseophagus fills up because the peristaltic waves cannot counter the backflow. Reflux is best demonstrated by first allowing the oesophagus to empty and then by rapidly rotating the infant a number of times. These manoeuvres are usually sufficient to demonstrate significant reflux, and it is unnecessary to go to such extremes as placing the infant in the Trendelenberg position. If there should be significant reflux a sliding hiatus hernia is probably present, and should be carefully looked for, and areas of ulceration, stricture, or persistent spasm should be recorded.

The elucidation of reflux on barium studies is difficult and exacting but the time spent on fluoroscopy must be limited to avoid undue chilling of the infant and unnecessary exposures to radiation. A diagnosis can usually be made within five to ten minutes and throughout the procedure the condition of the infant should be carefully watched; infants taken out of incubators are particularly liable to suffer from temperature changes.

Hiatus hernia

This term denotes a protrusion of the stomach through an abnormally wide oesophageal hiatus. In infants it is a congenital disease and may be demonstrated as early as the first week of life.

In the majority of cases the hernia remains small and no more than the bare area of the fundus of the stomach slides through the hiatus into the posterior mediastinum. There is no sac and the primary fault appears to be weakness and attenuation of the crural sling fibres which tend to regain their tone and bulk as the infant grows older. The cardia, however, is above the diaphragm and the main problem is reflux. The principal symptom is persistent vomiting, usually from birth. In general the vomiting is forceful and may be projectile. Peptic oesophagitis tends to occur and may be responsible for blood in the vomitus, the development of anaemia, and the development of a fibrous stricture of the oesophagus above the hernia. However, in most of the cases the symptoms tend to disappear at the age of about nine months.

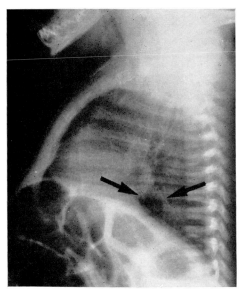

Figure 1.16. Small hiatus hernia (arrowed) seen in a lateral chest film

Figure 1.17. Small sliding hiatus hernia (arrow)

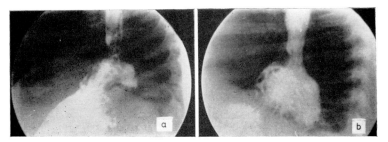

Figure 1.18. Sliding hiatus hernia in a month old infant, size variations occurred on crying

In about 25% of infants the hernia is large, with a considerable portion of the stomach protruding into the chest. In these cases a peritoneal hernial sac is present, situated in front of the stomach with extensions on each side. Some of these cases are simply an exaggeration of the small type described above. The cardia is well

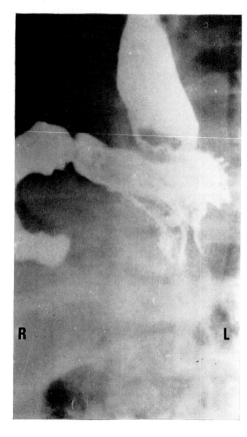

Figure 1.19a. Ten month old infant with a large para-oesophageal hernia; the stomach, which is partially filled, has herniated to the right

above the diaphragm and severe reflux with peptic oesophagitis is the main problem. The subsequent fibrosis which tends to extend widely into the wall of the oesophagus may result in severe strictures and permanent shortening of the oesophagus. (The vast majority, if not all, cases of so-called congenital short oesophagus are, in fact, cases of shortened oesophagus due to fibrosis following on peptic oesophagitis.)

Another variety of large hiatal hernia is sometimes referred to as a para-oesophageal hernia. In this type the hiatus is considerably enlarged due to almost complete absence of the diaphragmatic crus. The hernial sac tends to extend to the right of the oesophagus and may be a preformed congenital sac (perhaps persistent pneumato-enteric recess). The cardia may or may not rise above the level of the

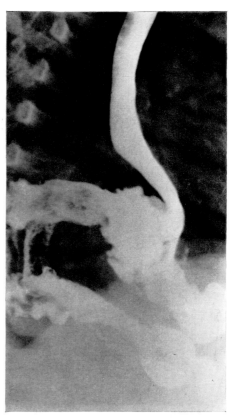

Figure 1.19b. Same case; the vestibule is in a relatively normal position but the majority of the stomach has herniated posteriorly

diaphragm but a loculus of the fundus of the stomach enters the hernia. As the hernia enlarges, more and more of the stomach moves up into the chest and in doing so is apt to rotate into the upside-down position. Sometimes the left lobe of the liver or the omentum, or even the transverse colon may enter the sac. (The condition is often confused with the parahiatal or rolling type of hernia found in

25

adults; in the latter condition, however, the herniation occurs through a defect in the crus and a narrow strip of muscle remains between the hernia and the oesophagus, while the cardia remains below the diaphragm.) This type of hernia tends to present later in infancy and childhood. Anaemia, as a result of bleeding into the thoracic loculus of the stomach from congested gastric veins, is the chief symptom and reflux is seldom a problem.

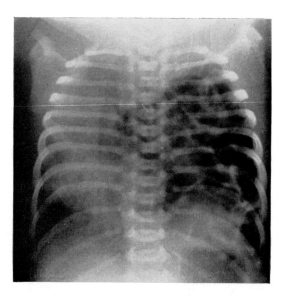

Figure 1.20. One day old infant with a left Bochdalek hernia

Radiological features

The diagnosis of hiatus hernia may be strongly suspected on clinical grounds, but is dependent on radiological recognition.

Plain films of the chest and abdomen may reveal air in a dilated oesophagus (*Figure 1.16*). This does not necessarily indicate an abnormality, but should raise the possibility of reflux. Occasionally an air-fluid level in an irreducible gastric loculus may be demonstrable.

Barium swallow is essential for a diagnosis, but may fail in small hernias, which tend to come and go, and repeated examinations may be necessary (*Figure 1.17*). Continuous free reflux is highly suggestive, but the crucial findings are the demonstrations of a vestibule above the diaphragm and/or a gastric loculus in the chest (*Figure 1.18*). Often the gastric mucosal rugae appear as characteristic ridges on the radiograph. In the para-oesophageal variety the oesophagus and cardia appear normal with the stomach rolled up alongside the oesophagus into the posterior mediastinum (*Figures 1.19a and b*). In all types, study of the playback videotapes or cineradiography will help to detect the presence of oesophagitis, ulceration, and strictures.

Diaphragmatic hernias

Congenital diaphragmatic hernia is one of the few extremely urgent emergencies in paediatric surgery where any delay in diagnosis and treatment may make all the difference between survival or death

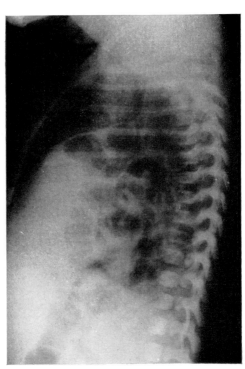

Figure 1.21. Lateral chest, Bochdalek hernia contained, to some degree, its sac

(4 of the 6 deaths in our last 26 cases could be attributed to delayed diagnosis). Prompt recognition is, therefore, of the utmost importance and depends upon both the clinician and the radiologist.

27

Embryology

The diaphragm is derived from several components. In the eighth week of foetal life the septum transversum develops in the cervical region of the embryo beneath the primitive heart and migrates dorsally to meet the mesentery of the foregut in the thoracolumbar region; this forms the central part of the diaphragm. Membranous

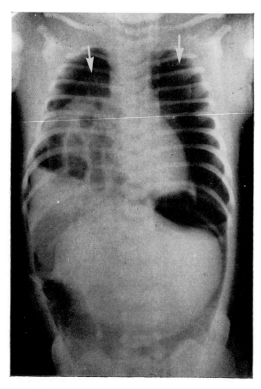

Figure 1.22. Two day old infant who was given forced ventilation for increasing respiratory distress; x-ray shows right Bochdalek hernia and bilateral pneumothoraces; gas has tracked down through the pleuroperitoneal canals into the abdomen

pleuroperitoneal folds then develop on each side and grow laterally and posteriorly to divide the peritoneal from the pleural cavity. Later, muscle fibres derived from the cervical myotomes grow between the peritoneal and pleural surfaces of these layers. The last portion to close is a triangular area situated posterolaterally and known as the foramen of Bochdalek, and the right side usually precedes the left. However, the formation of the diaphragm is complete by the end of the ninth week, i.e., just before the midgut starts returning from the 'physiological hernia' to the abdominal cavity (*see* Chapter 4).

Delayed closure of the diaphragm and improper muscular reinforcement lay the foundation for the common congenital abnormalities. Premature return of the midgut no doubt also plays a role and accounts for the frequent association of diaphragmatic hernias with anomalous rotation of the gut.

Failure of closure of the pleuroperitoneal folds will result in persistence of the pleuroperitoneal canal and a diaphragmatic hernia

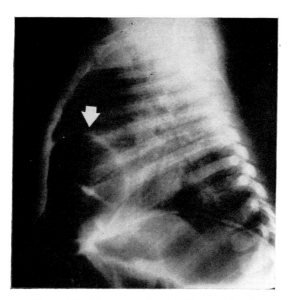

Figure 1.23. Chest x-ray showing Morgagni hernia

of the Bochdalek type without a peritoneal sac. However, if the folds have closed but are not adequately reinforced by invasion of muscle, the result will be a Bochdalek hernia with a sac, while complete failure of muscular reinforcement will result in eventration. Failure of fusion of the central and lateral portions of the diaphragm may also occur anteriorly leaving a defect known as the foramen of Morgagni. In most of these cases a sac is present and the fault is failure of muscular reinforcement.

Hernia through the foramen of Bochdalek

Persistence of the pleuroperitoneal canal with herniation of the abdominal contents into the pleural cavity is the hernia most commonly encountered in neonates. In about 80% of infants the hernia occurs on the left side and about 80% of the hernias have no peritoneal sac. The effects vary with the amount of bowel or other abdominal viscera (spleen, stomach, left lobe of liver) displaced into the pleural cavity, and the degree of displacement of the mediastinum or collapse of the lungs. Consequently hernias on the left and those with a sac tend to produce more urgent symptoms. On the right side

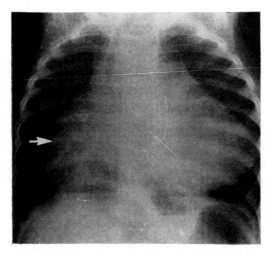

Figure 1.24a. Four week old infant with Fallot's tetralogy and a right lower mediastinal mass

the defect in the diaphragm is often plugged by the liver, which prevents other viscera from entering the chest, but small bowel and even stomach may herniate through the opening. Cyanosis, dyspnoea, and the rapid onset of respiratory distress are the classical symptoms. Sometimes the infant may seem normal at birth, but within a few hours, as the herniated bowel fills with gas, the symptoms develop and rapidly progress. Vomiting is an uncommon symptom and usually due to associated malrotation of the midgut.

On physical examination the outstanding features are severe tachypnoea with respiratory distresss, cyanosis, apparent dextrocardia in left-sided hernias, and a flat or scaphoid abdomen. Dullness to percussion and absence of respiratory sounds are additional findings, while the heart sounds are displaced to the opposite side. Peristaltic sounds are not usually heard.

Radiological features

Urgent and adequate radiology is essential for diagnosis. Plain films of the chest and abdomen will reveal the gas-filled intestinal loops in the affected side of the chest, displacement of the mediastinum to the opposite side and collapse of the lung, which occupies a small area at the apex of the pleural cavity (*Figures 1.20 and 1.21*). The abdomen is relatively airless because of absence of intestinal loops. Not infrequently there may be an associated pneumothorax of the opposite side and this should always be carefully looked for (*Figure 1.22*).

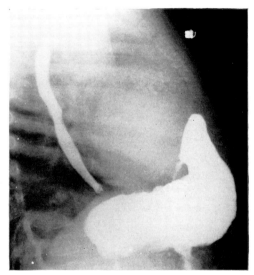

Figure 1.24b. Same case; barium meal demonstrating a Morgagni-type hernia

The radiological appearances are usually diagnostic, but in milder cases the bizarre pattern of bubbles in the chest may suggest, especially in right-sided hernias, staphylococcal pneumonia with pneumatocoele formation, or pyopneumothorax, and even congenital cystic disease of the lungs. In right-sided hernias where the defect is plugged by the liver, the latter may be sucked into the chest and present on the chest film as a dense rounded shadow. Contrast films are not required and, indeed, are contra-indicated in the acute cases presenting soon after birth. However, in smaller hernias with peritoneal sacs which may be surprisingly asymptomatic, contrast studies may be required later in life.

31

In the post-operative period expansion of the lungs must be checked on repeated films because the lung on the affected side, and even on the opposite side, may be hypoplastic. It is also important to look for evidence of pneumothorax on the contralateral side and for evidence of intestinal obstruction due to malrotation on the abdominal films.

Hernia through the foramen of Morgagni

Herniation through the anterior aspect of the diaphragm close to the sternocostal junction is much less common than that through the

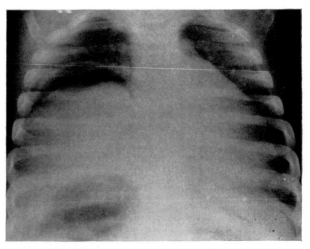

Figure 1.25. Right mediastinal mass, a small pneumoperitoneum showed liver below an eventration

foramen of Bochdalek. These hernias usually have a well-formed membranous sac which confines the herniating bowel and limits the degree of pulmonary compression or mediastinal displacement. Consequently, respiratory distress is unusual and most of the infants do not present in the neonatal period. Most commonly the transverse colon enters the sac with symptoms of partial large bowel obstruction; when the small bowel herniates through the foramen vomiting may be the first symptom.

The diagnosis may be suspected on routine plain films of the chest, especially on the lateral film, which may reveal a lower anterior mediastinal gas shadow (*Figure 1.23*). If, however, there is a mass not containing gas then contrast studies (barium meal and follow-through) are usually necessary (*Figures 1.24a and b*).

32

Eventration of the diaphragm

In this condition there is no defect in the diaphragm but the affected leaf is stretched out and weakened because of lack of muscular elements. Consequently the affected leaf rises high up into the pleural space compressing the affected lung.

Eventrations very rarely give rise to urgent symptoms and are not usually diagnosed in the neonatal period, but occasionally there may be respiratory distress.

Plain films will reveal the elevated leaf of the diaphragm rising into the pleural cavity with the abdominal organs lying below an arched line which separates the abdomen from the chest. On fluoroscopy paradoxical movements of the diaphragm may be seen. Sometimes a small pneumoperitoneum may be required to confirm the diagnosis and to exclude a mediastinal mass (*Figure 1.25*).

2

Plain Films of Abdomen

This chapter is devoted to general considerations in the examination of plain films of the abdomen. Further details on regional abnormalities will be found in the relevant chapters.

The plain film series, sometimes referred to as 'scout films', constitutes an important initial survey of the alimentary tract of any sick infant and must always be taken before contrast media are used. The series consists of three films taken in the supine, erect, and inverted lateral positions. The latter is often the most informative and should never be omitted. Further films are rarely necessary although lateral decubitus films may sometimes be of assistance.

It is important to have a systematic plan applicable to every film when the plain film series is viewed, and the following should be looked for on each film:

(1) Translucent air shadows, noting their quality, situation, and distribution; these normally require the most attention

(2) Soft tissue masses or fluid collections

(3) Calcific densities

(4) Skeletal abnormalities

AIR SHADOWS

Intra-abdominal air shadows are classified according to their situation in relation to the bowel, namely intraluminal, intramural, and extramural.

Intraluminal air shadows

Normal pattern

At birth the ability to swallow is well established and gas rapidly accumulates in the alimentary tract where its further propulsion is aided by deep respiratory movements which occur when the infant cries. Normally air reaches the large bowel by 3 hours and the whole alimentary tract is usually filled by 6 hours, but a delay in transit of up to 12 hours is still within the normal range. The normal air pattern consists of multiple, ill-defined, translucent areas which occupy the whole abdomen, excepting the right upper quadrant which contains the relatively large liver. A healthy infant

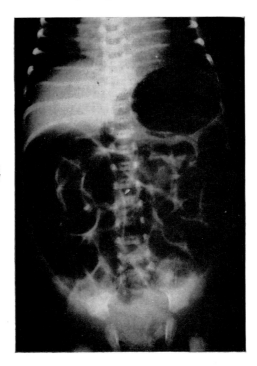

Figure 2.1. Normal gas pattern in a 24-hour old infant

usually has an abundant accumulation of air in the intestinal tract which is related to the amount of crying and time spent in the supine position.

The translucent air shadows within the bowel are relatively compressed so that a polyhedral pattern results, but the bowel is not unduly distended and no continuity of bowel loops is discernible (*Figure 2.1*). In the erect films occasional short air/fluid levels may be found. These are not necessarily significant, but in their evaluation it is important to correlate the radiological picture with the clinical findings.

35

Differentiation between large and small bowel may be very difficult. The watchspring appearance due to the plicae circulares of the small bowel and the interrupted haustral pattern of the large bowel, which can be seen in older children, are not evident in the neonate. Evaluation in terms of the anatomical situation of the colon is not reliable in the AP film. The inverted lateral film is likely to give most information; presence of air in the rectum indicates that gas

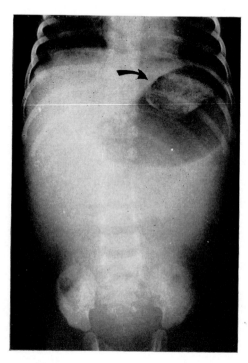

Figure 2.2. Relatively gasless abdomen in severe vomiting from gastroenteritis; the opacity in the stomach (arrowed) is from administered opaque medicament

has traversed the colon; the ascending and descending portions of the colon may sometimes be identified adjacent to the vertebral column, and gas in a dilated transverse colon may be seen extending forward toward the anterior abdominal wall. The value of this film in excluding mechanical obstruction is shown in *Figure 2.14.*

Abnormal air shadows

The abnormalities mainly concern the quantity and localization of the air and some of the illustrations will be found in the relevant chapters.

(a) *Excessive air shadows* are characteristic of intestinal obstruction. The distribution of air in the bowel is often best seen in a
supine film, while the erect and inverted lateral films will reveal the
presence of abnormal air/fluid levels if obstruction is present. The
inverted lateral film is particularly useful. Firstly, the presence of

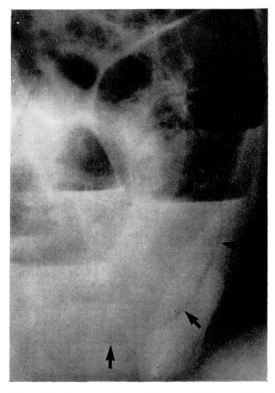

*Figure 2.3. Intra-mural gas (linear type) in necrotizing
enterocolitis*

air in the rectum rules out the possibility of intestinal atresia (rectal
examination or the insertion of a rectal thermometer introduces
only small amounts of air which may be responsible for no more
than a translucent sliver on the x-ray). Secondly, the situation of the
gas bubble is of particular value in the diagnosis of anorectal anomalies and will be discussed in Chapter 6.

Some obstructions have characteristic diagnostic patterns which will be discussed in the relevant sections. Amongst these, multiple fluid levels with distension of the bowel are particularly important because of the possibility of Hirschsprung's disease. It should also be borne in mind that excessive air/fluid levels are not always found in intestinal obstructions; for instance, in high intestinal obstructions and midgut volvulus there is a paucity of air/fluid levels, and in high obstructions there may even be complete absence of air.

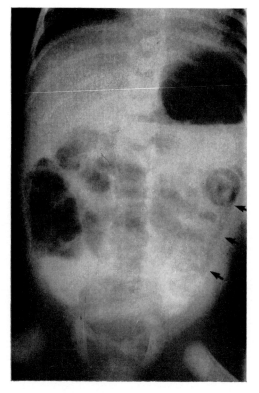

Figure 2.4. Intramural gas (cystic type) in necrotizing enterocolitis

(b) *Relative lack of air shadows*

(i) *High intestinal obstruction:* in the erect and inverted lateral films a few air/fluid levels will be present in grossly dilated bowel and this often indicates the site of the obstruction (*Figures 4.2, 4.6, 4.12*). Pyloric stenosis will usually show relatively few intestinal gas shadows (*Figure 3.2*).

(ii) *Midgut volvulus:* a relative paucity of air shadows with some fluid levels in a vomiting infant should always raise the possibility of midgut volvulus (*Figure 4.10*). The stomach is usually dilated.

(iii) *Diaphragmatic hernia:* the abdomen is relatively airless because the loops of bowel containing air have herniated into the thorax.

(iv) *Severe dehydration* caused by the vomiting and diarrhoea of gastroenteritis (*Figure 2.2*) or acute adreno-cortical insufficiency.

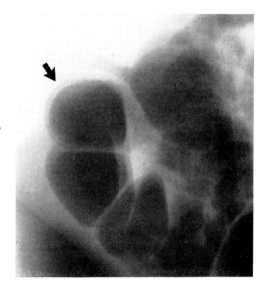

Figure 2.5. Intramural gas seen 'end on'

(v) *Infants who are unable to swallow air:* this applies particularly to patients suffering from tetanus neonatorum in whom tracheostomies have been performed. This is also the possible mechanism of the diminished gas shadows which may be seen in brain damaged infants or during the progression of hyaline membrane disease.

(vi) *Fluid in peritoneal cavity:* large amounts of fluid may reduce the amount of intestinal gas (see p. 47).

(c) *Complete absence of air shadows*

(i) Oesophageal atresia without a tracheo-oesophageal fistula (*Figure 1.6*).

(ii) High small bowel obstructions in which the stomach and bowel proximal to the obstruction are completely filled with fluid. In such cases a nasogastric tube should be passed, some of the fluid aspirated and replaced by air. The typical air/fluid levels of high intestinal obstruction will become obvious (*Figure 4.4*).

Intramural gas

Gas in the bowel wall shows up as a thin, radiotranslucent rim in the submucosal layer of the bowel (*Figure 2.3*); less frequently it has a cystic or bubbly appearance (*Figure 2.4*). It is often difficult to detect and may be seen only in one of the supine or erect films. Gas rims may sometimes be seen end-on as circular translucent areas at the margin of the bowel (*Figure 2.5*).

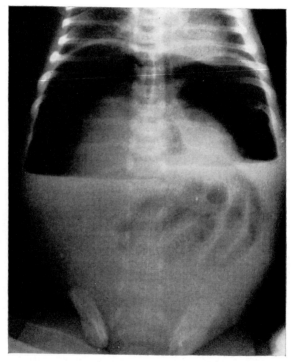

Figure 2.6. Pneumoperitoneum erect film, free fluid is also present

Intramural gas in infants bears no relation to the condition pneumatosis cystoides intestinalis seen in adults. It may be seen in the following conditions.

(a) *Necrotizing enterocolitis:* particularly in premature infants or less commonly following umbilical catheterization.

(b) *Hirschsprung's disease:* this is a debatable and minor feature, probably resulting from overdistension rather than a complicating enterocolitis (see p. 107).

(c) *Intestinal atresia,* as a rare incidental finding in the grossly distended proximal bowel.

The aetiology of the condition is obscure and will remain so until the nature and origin of the gas and the role played by gram negative bacteria are established. It is possible that selective circulatory ischaemia causes the initial necrosis in necrotizing enterocolitis. This may be the result of perinatal hypoxia in the premature infant or

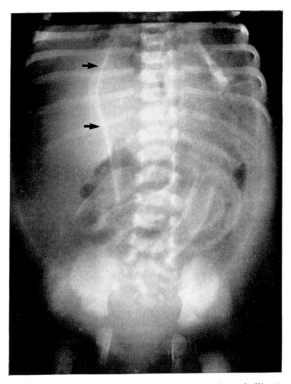

Figure 2.7. Pneumoperitoneum supine film. 'Football' sign with outlining of ligamentum teres; there is some thickening of the bowel walls from peritonitis

portal circulatory changes in the catheterized infant. In Hirschsprung's disease over-distension and stasis may cause a breach of the mucosal integrity and allow gas and organisms to enter the submucosa. Initially the gas may be no more than ectopic flatus but later it may be augmented by the action of gas-forming bacteria.

The gas tends to spread within the bowel wall and may rupture

into the peritoneal cavity causing pneumoperitoneum and peritonitis. Sometimes it enters the portal venous radicles and spreads to
the liver. Serial x-rays of the abdomen are necessary to detect these
complications.

Extramural gas

Pneumoperitoneum
    Free air in the peritoneal cavity shows up as a gas shadow under

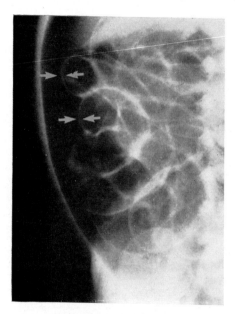

*Figure 2.8. Gas outlining
both sides of the bowel walls*

the diaphragm in the erect film. If excessive, it tends to push the liver
and spleen away from the diaphragm and the degree of separation
of these organs from the diaphragm usually indicates the degree of
pneumoperitoneum (*Figure 2.6*). In extreme cases air may even track
along a patent processus vaginalis into the scrotum.
    In the supine film the air will be seen underneath the anterior
abdominal wall in the shape of a dome tending to form a central,
oval translucent shadow. This collection of air is known as the
'football' sign. Frequently the falciform ligament is outlined by the
gas and shows as a curved, grey, opaque streak in the upper abdomen
(*Figure 2.7*). Occasionally even the urachus will be outlined in the

lower abdomen. Similarly, both sides of the bowel wall may be outlined by air. Normally only the inner surface of the bowel wall is outlined by intraluminal gas and the 'thickness' of the wall is, in fact, the combined shadow of the walls of two adjacent loops of bowel. When free air is present, however, the true thickness of the bowel wall is outlined by intraluminal air on the inside and free air

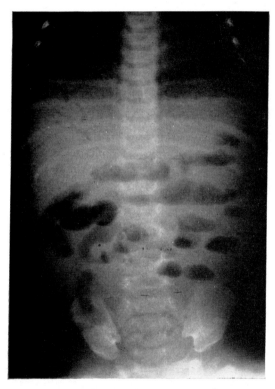

Figure 2.9. Gas in the portal vein in a case of necrotizing enterocolitis, the air shadows taper in a cephalad direction

on the outside (*Figure 2.8*). Pneumoperitoneum may result from perforations of the stomach, small bowel, or colon. The radiological and clinical features, however, are similar in all cases. Perforations of the stomach are three times as common as those of the small bowel, and are usually spontaneous. An indication of these cases is the absence of normal gas distension of the stomach. Small intestinal perforations are usually associated with obstructing lesions such as

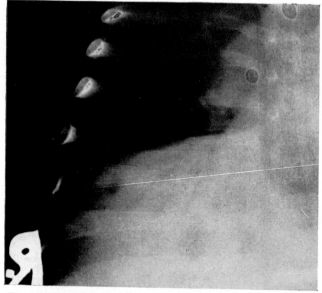

Figure 2.10. Bronchi distended by air seen in basal lung consolidation, the air shadows taper in a caudal direction

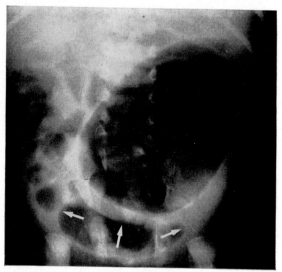

Figure 2.11. Gas in the bladder (arrows) (same case as Figure 4.7a)

44

atresias, but spontaneous or idiopathic types also occur in the terminal ileum. Colonic perforations usually occur in the caecal region and may be associated with necrotizing enterocolitis, Hirschsprung's disease, or strangulating volvulus. Pneumoperitoneum may also follow trauma by rectal catheters or thermometers. In this connection particular attention is drawn to the injudicious use of inflatable catheters for barium enemas in infants.

The presence of free air in a post-operative film should warn of the possibility of a leak or perforation. This is because air is not normally trapped in any quantity in the small space available.

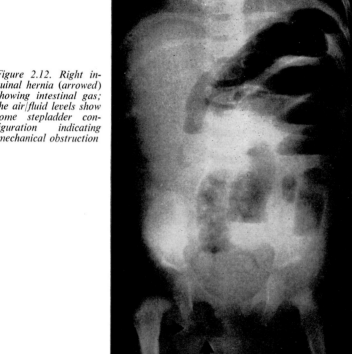

Figure 2.12. Right inguinal hernia (arrowed) showing intestinal gas; the air/fluid levels show some stepladder configuration indicating mechanical obstruction

Gas in the portal vein

This may occur in infants suffering from necrotizing enterocolitis (see pp. 40 and 106) and is a serious prognostic sign. The gas is recognized as thin, translucent lines radiating outwards in the liver area (*Figure 2.9*). These gas lines taper gradually in a cephalad direction.

They should be distinguished from air-filled bronchi in adjacent consolidated lung. In the latter, the translucent lines run obliquely downwards and taper in a caudal direction (*Figure 2.10*).

Gas in the urinary bladder (*Figure 2.11*)

The presence of gas in the urinary bladder is of particular importance in newborn infants suffering from anorectal malformations. It indicates a high or supralevator lesion with a fistula into the bladder, namely, anorectal agenesis with rectovesical fistula or sometimes the more common recto-urethral fistula (Chapter 6).

Extra-abdominal gas shadows

Bowel containing air may be visible in external hernias. *Figure 2.12* shows an inguinal hernia that is causing mechanical obstruction with a stepladder gas pattern.

SOFT TISSUE SHADOWS

Thickening of the bowel wall

This may be seen in inflammatory conditions of the bowel such as gastroenteritis and in severe cases is frequently associated with free fluid in the peritoneal cavity. In gastroenteritis there may also be multiple air/fluid levels resembling those of mechanical intestinal obstruction; thickening of the bowel wall is uncommon in the latter and, if present, suggests the diagnosis of gastroenteritis (*Figure 2.13*). However, gastroenteritis may be associated with paralytic ileus and then the air/fluid levels tend to be roughly in the same latitude when compared to the stepladder appearance of a mechanical obstruction (*Figure 2.12*). This may be difficult to evaluate and caution should be exercised in attempting to differentiate between gastroenteritis and mechanical obstructions. The inverted lateral film (*Figures 2.14a, b*) and the clinical history are the most helpful in diagnosis.

Free intraperitoneal fluid

The radiographic features of free fluid in the peritoneal cavity are:

(a) A generalized greyness or haziness of the abdomen.

(b) Frequently a paucity of gas shadows with thickening of the bowel wall.

(c) A 'frog-belly' appearance in the supine film due to the collection of fluid in the flanks while the intestinal gas shadows float upwards to the central position.

(d) Paucity of gas shadows in the lower abdomen in the erect film because the fluid gravitates to the pelvis while the intestinal gas shadows float upwards.

One of the common causes of free fluid in the newborn is urinary

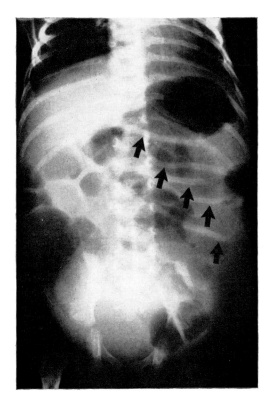

Figure 2.13. Thickened bowel wall (arrows) in severe gastroenteritis

ascites which may result from obstruction of the lower urinary tract, usually by posterior urethral valves. The obstruction causes a leakage or extravasation of urine from the kidneys, bladder, or ureters.

Another important cause of free fluid in the peritoneal cavity is intraperitoneal haemorrhage due to hypoprothrombinaemia associated with vitamin K deficiency. In such cases it may sometimes be possible to locate the source of the bleeding on the films by finding displacement of a gas-filled stomach or colon by blood which has collected at the bleeding site (*Figure 2.15*). Less common causes of free intraperitoneal fluid are portal hypertension due to posthepatic venous obstruction and chylous ascites. These conditions, however, usually do not occur until some weeks or months after birth.

Other masses

These appear as circumscribed areas of tissue density which may displace the gas shadows in adjacent bowel; the relative position of

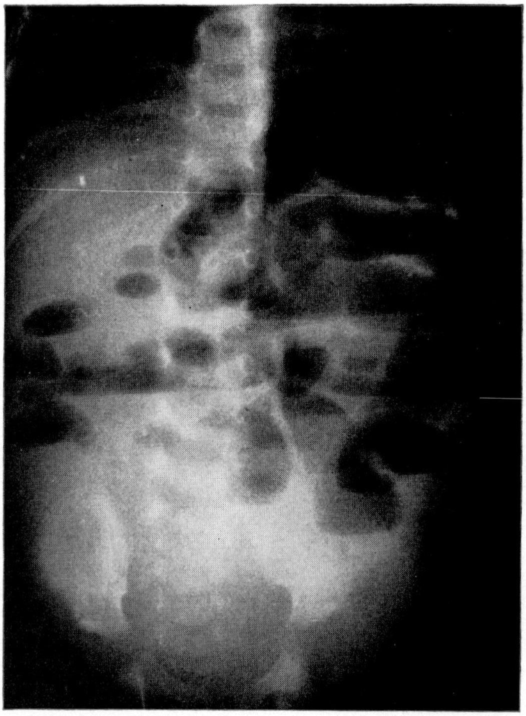

Figure 2.14a. Ileus, severe gastroenteritis in a month old infant; it is difficult to be certain whether this is mechanical or paralytic obstruction

the mass may indicate its site of origin. Masses in the upper abdomen may signify enlargement of the liver or spleen or a full, distended stomach. Masses in the loins are usually related to the kidney and, when unilateral, are commonly due to hydronephrosis, Wilms' tumour, neuroblastoma, or multicystic kidney. Central masses may be due to mesenteric cysts or intestinal duplications. Pelvic or lower

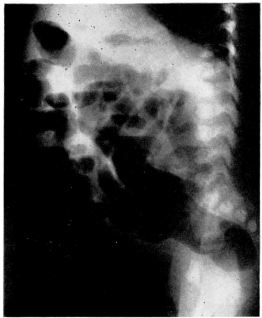

Figure 2.14b. Same case, inverted lateral film shows gas-distended rectum indicating that there is no gross mechanical obstruction

abdominal masses usually signify an enlarged bladder or a hydrocolpos, although both these organs may become so enlarged that their relative positions may be deceptive.

CALCIFIC DENSITIES

Meconium peritonitis causes diffuse streaks of calcification throughout the abdomen. The calcification may be extremely faint (*Figures 4.16, 4.17*), but is usually dense enough to outline the walls of the peritoneal cavity. In the typical case there is associated intestinal obstruction (see Chapter 4). Sometimes calcification may even extend along a patent processus vaginalis into the scrotum (*Figure 4.18*).

Calcification in the adrenal area is usually due to adrenal haemorrhage when it frequently appears as a fairly dense shadow (*Figure 2.16*). This should be differentiated from the fine, speckled calcification which sometimes occurs in neuroblastomas.

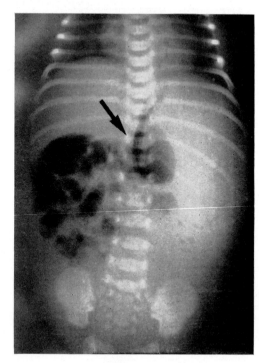

Figure 2.15. Haemoperitoneum in a 2-day-old infant, the central intestinal gas shadows and stomach (arrow) are displaced by a ruptured subcapsular haematoma of spleen

Figure 2.16 (below). Calcification of the right adrenal noted on the preliminary urogram film of a 3-week-old infant; the calcification was not evident in a further study seven months later

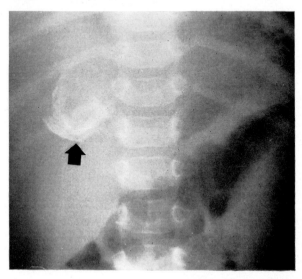

SKELETAL ABNORMALITIES

Vertebral abnormalities are common in infants suffering from ano-rectal malformations. The lumbosacral region is usually involved and the common abnormality is partial or complete absence of one or more sacral segments. Infants with high or supralevator lesions are more frequently affected, and in them the incidence of vertebral anomalies may be as high as 30–40%.

Hemivertebrae may also occur in association with neuroenteric cysts and are usually seen in the cervical or upper dorsal spine. They constitute part of the split notochord syndrome (*Figure 1.9*).

Bony abnormalities unassociated with abnormalities of the alimentary tract may also be seen, for instance, an unsuspected dislocation of the hip or metaphyseal translucencies and periosteal layering due to congenital syphilis (this condition is still prevalent in some parts of the world).

3

The Stomach

The stomach of a normal neonate lies on a more transverse or horizontal plane than that of the older child in whom the erect posture brings about the adult J-shape. The pyloric canal and duodenal bulb are not seen in the direct AP view because they are situated posteriorly and cephalad behind the pyloric antrum. The pyloric canal is, therefore, best visualized in the prone oblique (almost lateral) position. The gastric rugae have a smooth appearance although the mucosa may be seen puckered into a star-shaped configuration at the inner aspect of the cardia.

Persistent vomiting is the usual reason for performing a contrast examination of the stomach of a newborn baby. Frequently, the patient is referred with a provisional clinical diagnosis of oesophageal reflux, hiatus hernia, or pyloric stenosis. The following method of examination is recommended to avoid the administration of too much barium which might obscure the pathology.

(a) The baby is turned into the prone position and allowed to suck a limited amount of dilute barium from a feeding bottle. Only a brief glance at the oesophagus is taken at this stage because the pylorus should be examined first for evidence of pyloric stenosis.

(b) The duodenum is then examined for possible stenosis or obstructing bands associated with malrotation.

(c) Then more barium is given and the lower end of the oesophagus examined. We prefer initial visualization in the prone position to study the peristalsis of the lower end of the oesophagus. The baby is then turned into the supine position and rotated a number of times to allow barium to pool at the cardia. If no organic lesion is found the vomiting may be due to feeding problems, infections or neurological disturbances such as meningitis or birth trauma. Adrenal hyperplasia, which may cause projectile vomiting, and severe salt deficiency should be borne in mind, particularly if ambiguous genitalia are present.

CONGENITAL HYPERTROPHIC PYLORIC STENOSIS

Pyloric stenosis is a common condition with an incidence which varies from 1 in 300 to 1 in 900 live births in Western countries. The

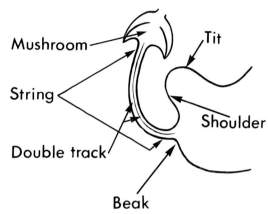

Figure 3.1. Diagrammatic representation of the contrast meal features of pyloric stenosis

male:female ratio is 5:1 and firstborn infants are more commonly affected than others.

Clinical presentation

The presenting symptom is vomiting of gastric content which is not bile-stained. It usually begins in the third or fourth week of life, but may occur at any time from birth to the age of five months. In a series of 165 cases seen at the Red Cross Children's Hospital during the period 1956–1967, 30% of the infants presented between the third and fourth weeks but a significant number (6%) presented in the first week of life. The condition was uncommon in African infants. Initially the vomiting may be little more than a regurgitation after the feed, but soon it becomes forceful and projectile. When vomiting has been prolonged and severe, dehydration and alkalosis ensue and the vomitus may contain coffee-ground material due to superadded gastritis.

'Golf ball' peristalsis may be seen in the epigastrium passing from

53

left to right and a pyloric tumour is usually palpable—in the series referred to above a tumour was palpable in 83% of the cases. The average tumour is smooth, 2 to 3 cm long, oval shaped, and usually situated slightly to the right of the midline in the epigastrium. It is often better felt immediately after the baby has vomited or the stomach emptied by nasogastric aspiration. If a tumour is palpable by examination a barium meal is unnecessary and should not be carried out.

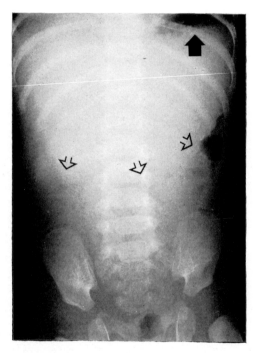

Figure 3.2. Pyloric steno-sis erect film; the fluid level (solid arrow) is present in a grossly dilated stomach (arrowheads); there is little gas in the rest of the in-testines

Radiology

We have found that the plain films may provide valuable and consistent information. In the erect film the fluid-distended stomach extending to approximately the level of L4 can be visualized, while the air/fluid level in the fundus of the stomach is situated high up in the left upper quadrant, and there is a relative paucity of gas in the intestines (*Figure 3.1*). The supine film often reveals the ventral surface of the distended stomach outlined by air, and a constricting

wave of peristalsis may sometimes be seen (*Figure 3.2*). These findings are highly suggestive of pyloric stenosis and, if present, should
prompt further efforts at finding a palpable tumour.

If a contrast meal should be necessary, a 50% W/V solution of
barium should be used and given by feeding bottle in small amounts.
If a large amount of retained fluid is present in the stomach it should

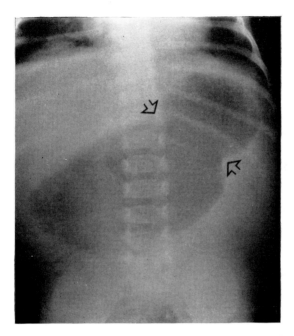

*Figure 3.3. Plain film of pyloric stenosis; a 'golf ball' wave of
peristalsis is arrowed*

be aspirated through a nasogastric tube, after which the investigation
can be carried out by injecting small amounts of barium through the
tube. Fluoroscopy should be carried out with the baby in the prone
oblique-lateral position when the narrow pyloric canal may be seen
curving upwards and to the left. In the early stages when barium
has filled only the pyloric antrum, the canal is often poorly outlined
and can be better seen by rotating the baby laterally to allow visualization of the canal through the air-filled fundus.

The pylorus of a normal newborn baby opens within five to ten
minutes of the commencement of the examination, but when pyloric

stenosis is present a delay of thirty minutes and more is not uncommon. If no barium has passed through the pylorus after thirty
minutes it is futile to continue the examination.

The radiological diagnosis is made on the following features
(*Figures 3.3, 3.4, 3.5*):

(a) A 'beak' at the commencement of the pyloric canal

(b) The 'string' of the narrowed pyloric canal which curves up
and to the left

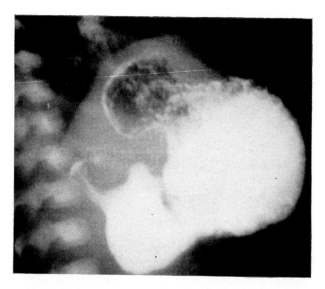

Figure 3.4. Pyloric stenosis

(c) A 'mushroom' where the pyloric tumour indents the base of
the duodenal cap

(d) Sometimes a 'double track' in the pyloric canal due to infold-
ing of the mucosa

(e) The 'tit' due to the persistence of a peristaltic wave on the
lesser curvature protruding upwards like a small breast

(f) The 'shoulder' due to adjoining tumour on the lower concave
border of the 'tit'

The 'string' and 'beak' appearances together may look like an
umbrella with a bent handle.

These radiological appearances may persist post-operatively for
several months, even though the stenosis has been clinically relieved.

56

Pylorospasm or failure of relaxation of the pyloric region may be difficult to differentiate from pyloric stenosis. The narrowing, however, is not constant in appearance and apart from the 'beaking' and narrowing of the canal, the features that have been noted above are not consistently present.

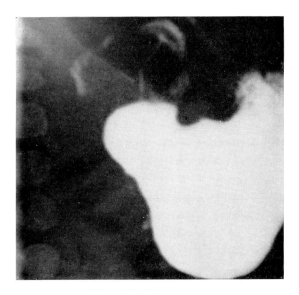

Figure 3.5. Pyloric stenosis

UNCOMMON CONDITIONS

Pyloric membrane

This membrane consists of a web of normal gastric mucosa situated in the pyloric canal and may be complete or have a central aperture. A correct pre-operative diagnosis is not common, but can be made on barium meal if there is an obstruction in the region of the pyloric canal without the features of a pyloric tumour (*Figure 3.6*).

Microgastria

In this condition there is hypoplasia of the stomach which may be associated with other visceral or skeletal abnormalities. A small

57

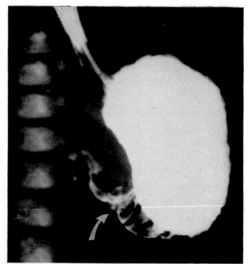

Figure 3.6. Pyloric membrane (arrow)

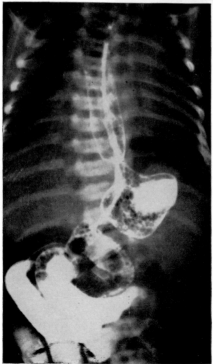

Figure 3.7. Microgastria (courtesy Dr. H. Kaufmann, Philadelphia)

stomach is demonstrable on barium meal and there is frequently associated oesophageal reflux (*Figure 3.7*).

Duplication cysts

These occur on the greater curvature of the stomach and, though sharing a common muscular wall, do not usually communicate with

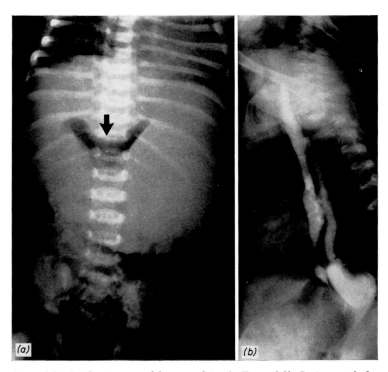

(a)

(b)

Figure 3.8a. Duplication cyst of the stomach in a 9-day old infant; gas in the normal stomach is arrowed (courtesy Dr. J. Moir, St. John N.B., J. Can. Assoc. Rad.)

Figure 3.8b. Barium meal after a window had been created between the stomach and cyst; there is now free reflux from the re-duplicated stomach into the blind ended oesophagus

the gastric lumen, but fill with fluid to form a mass which may compress the stomach (*Figure 3.8a*). Sometimes these cysts are associated with duplication of the oesophagus (*Figure 3.8b*). The inner lining of the cyst consists of gastric mucosa and a Technetium scan may be of help in the diagnosis.

59

Perforation of the stomach

Perforation of the stomach is a common cause of sudden abdominal distension and pneumoperitoneum in the newborn. The aetiology of the condition is uncertain but the infants are frequently premature. Defects of the gastric musculature, perforation

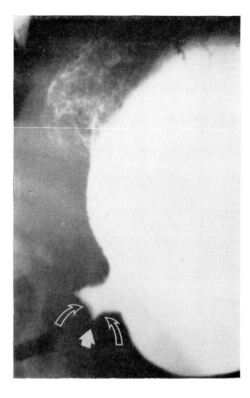

Figure 3.9. One year old infant with ulcer (arrow); the oedematous shoulders (curved arrows) are causing pyloric obstruction (referred with diagnosis of pyloric stenosis)

by a nasogastric tube, infection, and localized ischaemic necrosis have all been implicated.

Tumours

Gastric tumours are exceedingly rare in the newborn but teratomas have been reported.

Ulcers

Gastric ulcers or erosions may occur in the newborn and be

responsible for bleeding or perforation. They are likely to be associated with prematurity or brain damage. These ulcers are not radiologically demonstrable as they form shallow erosions unassociated with the niche or scarring seen in adults. However, later in childhood a typical niche may be seen. Childhood ulcers are usually acute and surrounded by oedema and this may cause obstruction to the pylorus (*Figure 3.9*)

Torsion of the stomach

Spontaneous, axial torsion of the stomach without associated diaphragmatic defects is an extremely rare cause of vomiting in the newborn. The radiological features in the supine position, however, are characteristic. The body of the stomach is at a higher level than normal with the greater curve cephalad and the lesser curve caudad.

4

Small Intestine

Abnormalities of the small bowel in the neonate are predominantly congenital in nature and the majority present with symptoms and signs of intestinal obstruction, namely vomiting, distension and constipation.

Vomiting, particularly when it is persistent and bile-stained, is a most important warning symptom and should always raise the possibility of a mechanical intestinal obstruction.

Abdominal distension is variable and depends on the level of the obstruction. It may be minimal in duodenal and proximal jejunal obstruction but is usually considerable with obstructions in the lower small bowel. Sometimes the distended loops may be seen and visible peristalsis may be evident.

Constipation is the least informative symptom. In normal infants meconium is usually evacuated on the first day of life, changing to milk stools by the third day. In infants with intestinal obstruction there may be absolute constipation but frequently a small amount of meconium, which was present in the bowel distal to the obstruction, is passed on the first and second days of life. In incomplete obstructions and those proximal to the ampulla of Vater the baby may continue to pass larger quantities of meconium.

High intestinal obstructions are associated with signs of dehydration, the degree of which will depend on the length of the history and the severity of the vomiting. Jaundice is also a frequent finding. In low obstructions dehydration may also be severe and if there is associated strangulation there will be signs of toxaemia.

A clinical diagnosis of obstruction will be confirmed by the plain film series which will usually reveal dilated gas-filled loops of bowel and fluid levels. In addition, the x-rays may also indicate the site of the obstruction.

When the plain films confirm the presence of obstruction it is our policy to do a contrast enema for the following reasons:

(a) It is difficult and sometimes impossible to differentiate obstructed lower small bowel from obstructed large bowel (see Chapter 5).

(b) The presence of a microcolon, i.e., an unused colon, is diagnostic of small bowel atresia or meconium ileus.

(c) Large bowel pathology can be excluded. This applies particularly to an associated colonic atresia which might otherwise be missed, even at operation.

(d) Rotational abnormalities can be detected from the position of the caecum. These may be the cause of the obstruction and are also frequently associated with small bowel atresia.

The details of the technique of contrast enemas and interpretation of the films are discussed in Chapter 5.

A contrast meal is contra-indicated in most obstructive lesions because of the danger of regurgitation and aspiration. However, a contrast meal may be useful and justifiable if partial duodenal obstruction is suspected. In such cases a small amount of contrast material should be injected through an intragastric tube, to minimize the risk of aspiration. After the examination the contrast media should be withdrawn to prevent inspissation of barium in the bowel.

The main causes of obstruction in the small bowel are:

(a) *Duodenum*
    (i) Atresia and stenosis
    (ii) Annular pancreas (an uncommon lesion)
    (iii) Rotational anomalies

(b) *Small intestine*
    (i) Atresia and stenosis
    (ii) Meconium ileus
    (iii) Meconium peritonitis
    (iv) Functional obstruction
    (v) Miscellaneous, including duplications, internal or external hernias, intussusception, and Hirschsprung's disease.

DUODENAL OBSTRUCTIONS

Atresia and stenosis

Intrinsic duodenal obstruction occurs once in approximately ten thousand births, and 60% of the infants are premature. In approximately 30% of cases the obstruction is proximal to the ampulla of Vater. The various types that occur are (*Figure 4.1*):

(a) A blind-ending dilated proximal pouch with a distal collapsed segment in continuity, i.e., a membranous obstruction

(b) A blind-ending proximal dilated pouch disconnected from the collapsed distal segment

(c) A proximal blind-ending dilated pouch connected to the distal collapsed bowel by a fibrous band

(d) Duodenal stenosis or an incomplete diaphragm

(e) Duodenal stenosis with bile duct entering the stenosed area

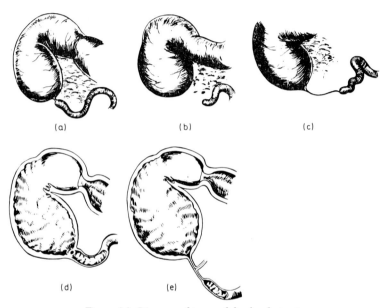

(a)   (b)   (c)

(d)   (e)

Figure 4.1. Diagram of types of duodenal atresia

Atresia and stenosis of the duodenum are probably due to failure of recanalization of the solid stage of the duodenum and not to a vascular accident, as in the case of more distal atresias. About 30% of the patients suffer from Down's syndrome. This can be detected on the pelvis x-ray by measuring the iliac index which is the sum of the acetabular and iliac angles; in Mongolism it is in the region of 60°. Annular pancreas and malrotation of the intestine are also commonly associated with duodenal atresia and stenosis. Other associated abnormalities include atresias of the oesophagus and distal small bowel and congenital abnormalities of the anorectal region, heart, and urinary tract.

Clinical features

Persistent vomiting is the cardinal sign of duodenal obstruction. The vomiting is bile-stained in infra-ampullary obstructions and clear but persistent in supra-ampullary lesions. The degree of de-

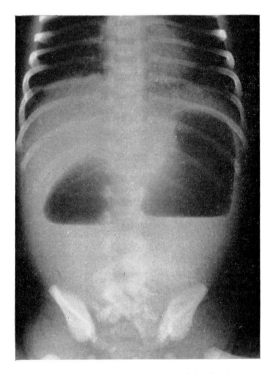

Figure 4.2. Classical 'double bubble' of duodenal atresia

hydration of the infant will depend on the length of delay before the diagnosis is made. Maternal hydramnios is a common feature.

Radiological features

In duodenal atresia the erect film usually reveals a classical 'double bubble' (*Figure 4.2*) due to air/fluid levels in the dilated stomach and first part of the duodenum. If the obstruction is in the distal duodenum there may even be a 'treble bubble' appearance (*Figure 4.3*). However, if the duodenum and stomach are filled with fluid there may be no air/fluid levels. In such cases the gastric contents

65

should be aspirated and a small amount of air injected through a nasogastric tube when the abnormal pathology will present (*Figure 4.4*).

Rarer features are gas in the stomach wall when there is gross distension and even a few tiny spots of gas distal to the obstruction if a bifid hepatopancreatic duct is present.

A contrast enema is not necessary when the diagnosis is obvious on the plain x-rays. However, if it should be performed a narrow,

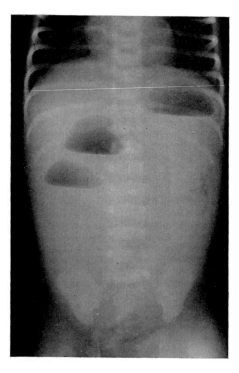

Figure 4.3. A 'treble bubble' appearance; this was a case of distal duodenal atresia with a malrotation of the duodenum; appearances would also be consistent with high jejunal atresia

unused 'microcolon' will usually be demonstrated, except when the obstruction is supra-ampullary, in which case the colon may be normally distended due to the passage of biliary and pancreatic secretions (*Figure 4.5*).

In duodenal stenosis a 'double bubble' may or may not be seen depending on the severity of the obstruction. Furthermore, small quantities of gas will be visible in the distal bowel (*Figure 4.6*). In the membranous type of stenosis the obstructing membrane tends to bulge well down into the distal duodenum (windsock deformity), thus giving a wrong impression of the exact site of the obstruction. Not infrequently it may be necessary to inject air or a small amount of barium down a nasogastric tube to confirm the diagnosis of duodenal stenosis (*Figure 4.7*).

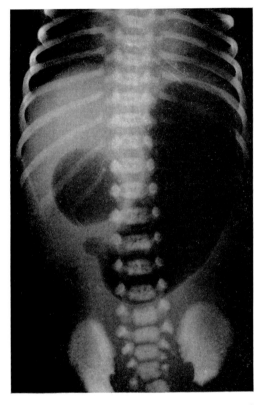

Figure 4.4. Duodenal atresia demonstrated by stomach aspiration and injection of air

Annular pancreas

In this condition the head of the pancreas encircles the second part of the duodenum to a variable extent giving rise to a variable degree of duodenal obstruction. It is rarely encountered as an isolated lesion in newborn infants and is usually associated with duodenal stenosis and atresia. In older infants, however, it may occur

67

as an isolated lesion, in which the clinical and radiological features are similar to those of duodenal stenosis.

Rotational anomalies

An understanding of the normal rotation of the foetal gut is necessary to appreciate rotational anomalies. In the earliest days of de-

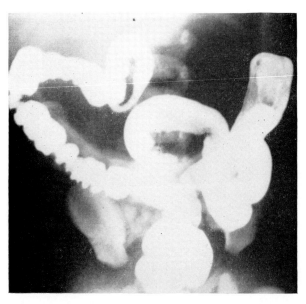

Figure 4.5. Supra-ampullary duodenal atresia; barium enema showed that there is no microcolon because bile and pancreatic ducts enter below the atresia; note the high midline position of caecum and appendix indicating a malrotation

velopment the alimentary canal is represented by a tube suspended in the midline of the abdominal cavity by a ventral and dorsal mesentery. It consists of three portions, foregut, midgut, and hindgut, each of which has its own artery. Departures from the normal situation of the derivations of the foregut and hindgut are exceedingly rare. Errors in the location of the alimentary canal are therefore almost entirely confined to the midgut loop, which extends from the ampulla of Vater to the junction of the middle and left third of the transverse colon.

The primitive midgut, which is supplied by the superior mesenteric artery, forms a loop convex forward. It grows so rapidly that the coelomic cavity is too small to hold it, and part of the loop is extruded into the extra-embryonic coelom or physiological hernia in the umbilical cord, with the artery running from the aorta through the duodeno-colic isthmus to the apex of the extruded gut. The mid-

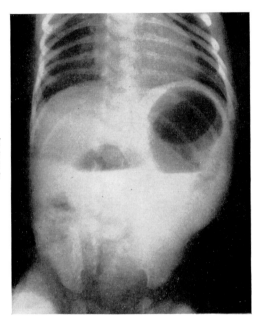

Figure 4.6. Duodenal stenosis; a 'double bubble' appearance with some distal intestinal gas

gut loop and mesentery still lie in the sagittal plane. The part cephalad to the artery is the prearterial segment (*Figure 4.8a*).

The first stage of rotation occurs while the loop lies in the umbilical cord between the fifth and tenth weeks. It is largely brought about by the great growth of the right lobe of the liver downwards and to the right, which exercises pressure on the prearterial segment of the midgut loop pushing it down and to the right. The movement of the prearterial segment forces the postarterial segment upwards and to the left, and thus completes the first stage of rotation. The growth of the liver has thus succeeded in rotating the midgut loop through 90° in an anticlockwise direction.

The second stage of rotation commences in the tenth week when the midgut starts returning to the abdominal cavity from the umbilical cord. The prearterial segment returns first and while this occurs, the superior mesenteric artery remains fixed to the umbilicus and stretched like a cord from commencement to termination. The returning small gut enters the abdomen to the right of the artery but, the space there being limited, the coils are pushed to the left behind the taut artery, and in doing so, they displace the hindgut

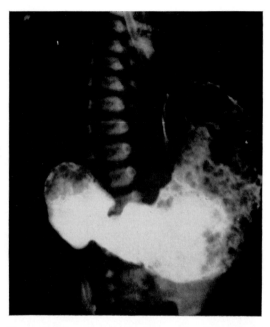

Figure 4.7. Complete duodenal obstruction demonstrated by a limited contrast meal administered by an oesophageal tube

before them so that the descending colon comes to occupy the left flank. The last coil of ileum carries the superior mesenteric artery with it as it is reduced. The postarterial segment, i.e., caecum and ascending colon, then reduces, passing upwards to the right and crossing the pedicle of the small gut close to the origin of the superior mesenteric artery. The caecum, therefore, comes to lie under the liver but, with subsequent growth and elongation of the colon, is pushed into the right loin. This completes the second stage of rotation. It should be noted that by this time the midgut loop has rotated through 270° from its original sagittal plane; that the

70

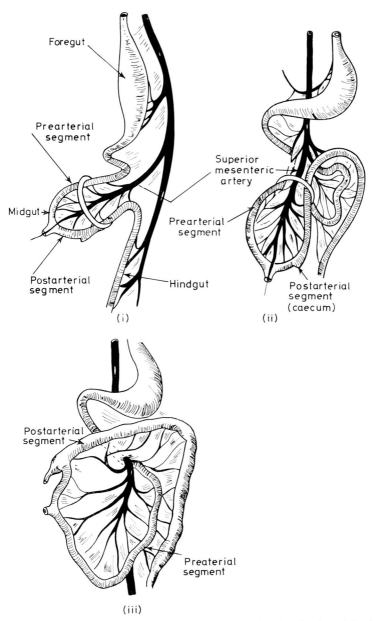

Figure 4.8a. Normal rotation of foetal intestines: (i) fifth foetal week: the umbilical hernia of midgut, just prior to rotation; (ii) tenth foetal week: end of first stage of rotation (90°); the prearterial segment is about to return beneath the superior mesenteric artery to the left upper coelomic cavity; (iii) eleventh foetal week: end of second stage of rotation (a further 180°); the whole of the midgut has returned and the caecum will descend further prior to fixation

duodenum crosses behind the superior mesenteric artery and the transverse colon in front of it; that the descending colon occupies the left flank; and that the caecum is in the right loin.

The third stage is concerned mainly with the firm fixation of the

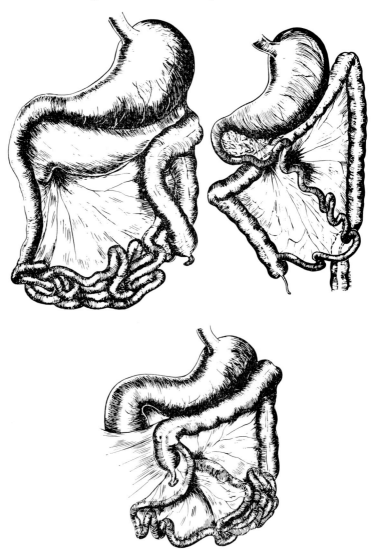

Figure 4.8b. Diagram of the types of rotational abnormalities

gut to the posterior abdominal wall, but before this occurs, the caecum descends further to reach the right iliac fossa.

The process of rotation may be arrested at any stage or, less commonly, may deviate from the normal routine resulting in several anomalies, the most important of which are:

Persistence of the first stage of rotation

This is very rare but may occur in some cases of omphalocoele. The small and large bowel have a common longitudinal mesentery with virtually no rotation.

Derangement of the second stage of rotation (*Figure 4.8b*)

(a) *Non-rotation of the midgut loop:* in this condition the duodenum descends from its normal fixed upper part down along the right side of the superior mesenteric artery, the small gut lies chiefly to the right of the midline, and the colon is confined to the left side of the abdomen. This disposition of the gut is usually associated with lack of fixation so that the whole midgut loop is suspended by an extremely narrow pedicle. The condition is relatively rare and it usually causes no symptoms but may predispose to volvulus.

(b) *Reversed rotation of the midgut loop:* the transverse colon crosses behind the superior mesenteric artery while the duodenum crosses in front of it. Otherwise the intestines are in their normal position but lack of fixation is common. This rare anomaly seldom causes symptoms but may also predispose to volvulus.

(c) *Malrotation of the midgut loop* implies irregular defects of rotation during the second stage and includes a number of variants. Usually rotation has been arrested towards the end of the second stage, i.e., the caecum fails to descend and lies anterior to the duodenum where it becomes fixed by bands which cross the duodenum to emerge with the posterior parietal peritoneum in the right upper quadrant. These bands obstruct the second part of the duodenum to a variable degree. There is often associated non-fixation of the mesentery with a tendency to midgut volvulus. This condition is common and is often referred to as Ladd's syndrome.

Derangement of the third stage of rotation

(a) Failure of fixation often accompanies other rotational anomalies but may exist by itself. In such cases the caecum has descended to the right iliac fossa and the right colon is suspended on a long, mobile mesentery. This anomaly, which is comparatively common, predisposes to midgut or caecal volvulus and also to intussusception.

(b) Rarely, excessive fixation may occur in the region of the third and fourth parts of the duodenum with a variable degree of compression of the bowel.

In summary, it should be noted that rotational anomalies tend to cause duodenal obstruction in one of two ways. Firstly by abnormal bands of fixation which run from a misplaced caecum across the duodenal loop, and secondly from a lack of fixation which predisposes to a volvulus of the midgut. When the latter occurs the bowel

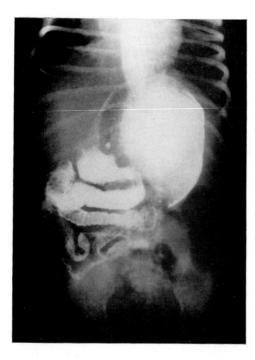

Figure 4.9. Limited gastrografin meal showing dilated stomach in a case of Ladd's bands; further views showed a dilated duodenum, but this one is selected to show the relatively collapsed malrotated small intestine

is secondarily obstructed at the duodenojejunal junction and in addition there is a great risk of midgut infarction. Because of the seriousness of the latter complication, the possibility of volvulus should always be borne in mind if rotational anomalies are suspected.

Clinical features

Bile-stained vomiting is the presenting feature but may not occur in the first two or three days of life and meconium may be passed normally. When the condition is complicated by midgut volvulus the symptoms tend to be more acute, and if intestinal strangulation has occurred some blood may be passed per rectum or a coffee-ground aspirate may be obtained from the stomach.

Abdominal distension is not a prominent feature, except in some of the cases when complicated by midgut volvulus. In some infants the symptoms of obstruction may subside only to recur after days or weeks.

Radiological features

Plain films may show a distended stomach and dilated proximal

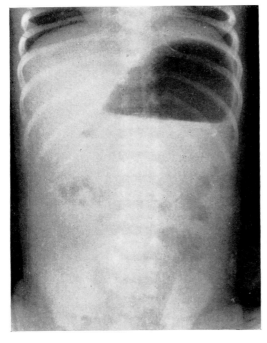

Figure 4.10. Midgut volvulus; there is a distended stomach with only a few centrally placed gas shadows. On some occasions these gas shadows will be more distended

duodenum with air/fluid levels similar to those of duodenal atresia or stenosis. Since the obstruction is incomplete some gas will be present in the distal bowel. In doubtful cases obstruction due to Ladd's bands can be demonstrated by injecting a small amount of barium down a nasogastric tube (*Figure 4.9*).

Complicating midgut volvulus should be suspected when there

75

is a paucity of gas shadows in the abdomen associated with a dilated stomach and sometimes air/fluid levels in centrally placed gut (*Figure 4.10*). The possibility of this condition should always be borne in mind when assessing the plain x-rays of any vomiting infant, especially when the vomit is bile-stained. In such cases early diagnosis is of paramount importance to anticipate the serious complication of infarction, and can be made by means of a contrast enema.

Details of the enema technique are given in Chapter 5. When there is deviation of the mid-transverse colon, malrotation can be diagnosed, and when the ascending colon is involved or obstructed, complicating midgut volvulus has most probably occurred. To avoid overfilling of the colon it is essential to stop injecting contrast when the transverse colon commences to fill and to inject in gradual stages thereafter. A normally placed caecum which cannot be displaced usually excludes a malrotation. It may, however, be difficult to decide if a caecum, which appears a little high in position, is malrotated. On the other hand, a caecum which is subhepatic or situated in the midline should be considered abnormal.

SMALL BOWEL OBSTRUCTION

Atresia and stenosis of the jejunum and ileum

One newborn baby in approximately every three thousand suffers from intestinal atresia or stenosis. The ileum is most commonly affected and in approximately 10% of cases there are multiple areas of atresia.

There are four types of intrinsic occlusion of the small bowel (*Figure 4.11*).

(a) *Stenosis:* there is a zone of narrowing of the intestinal lumen which, in many cases, will barely admit a probe.

(b) *Atresia type 1:* one or more septa or diaphragms completely occlude the lumen. These septa may contain all the intestinal layers in duplicate, but more frequently there are only a few muscle fibres or simply two layers of mucosa.

(c) *Atresia type 2:* the proximal bowel terminates in a blind end and the distal bowel commences similarly, the two ends being joined by a fibrous band. The adjoining mesentery may be intact, or there may be a V-shaped defect corresponding to the atretic segment.

(d) *Atresia type 3:* the proximal and distal blind ends are completely separated with no connecting band. The total length of the small bowel may be considerably reduced. The adjoining mesentery always has a V-shaped defect corresponding to the missing segment.

Unlike patients suffering from duodenal occlusions, infants with jejuno-ileal lesions seldom have associated serious anomalies of other systems, and Mongolism is a rarity. However, inadequate fixation of the bowel is common, and jejuno-ileal atresias have been encountered in cases with meconium ileus and occur in approximately 3% of infants with omphalocoele or gastroschisis.

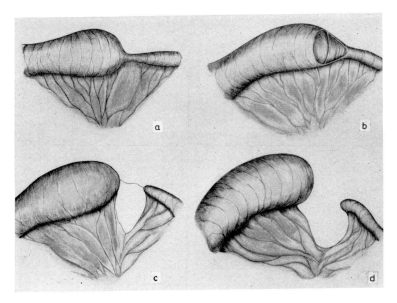

Figure 4.11. Diagram of types of intestinal atresia

Pathogenesis

It is now generally accepted that intestinal atresia and stenosis below the duodenum are caused by an intra-abdominal vascular accident during intra-uterine life. This results not merely in arrest of growth but in actual disappearance of the affected portion of the foetal bowel.

Clinical features

Bile-stained vomiting is the presenting symptom and the higher the obstruction the earlier the vomiting. The onset of bile-stained vomiting may be delayed in intestinal stenosis.

Abdominal distension is often present, being less marked in the high and incomplete obstructions.

Constipation is not absolute until the meconium present in the bowel distal to the obstruction has been evacuated. This amount is not large and it is not sufficient to dilate the unused colon (microcolon). Consequently the findings on rectal examination are often misinterpreted as those of a rectal anomaly.

Radiological features

The diagnosis is usually apparent on the plain films. A jejunal atresia will have comparatively few dilated intestinal loops (*Figures 4.12a, b*), but there is always the possibility that these will be fluid-filled, giving a gasless abdomen. In cases of doubt, aspiration and insufflation of air should be carried out. Ileal atresia will show more

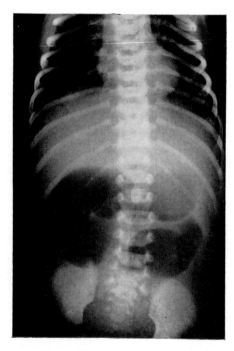

Figure 4.12a. Supine film of jejunal atresia

distended loops of bowel with multiple fluid levels (*Figure 4.13*). These are usually of approximately the same dilated calibre with the exception of the most distal loop, which may be grossly dilated. It is these low intestinal obstructions which are difficult to differentiate from colonic obstruction and they require a contrast enema to show the microcolon of small bowel atresia or the associated malrotation that predisposed to the infarction in utero.

Meconium ileus

In meconium ileus the terminal ileum is obstructed by masses of abnormal meconium. It is the earliest manifestation of mucoviscidosis or cystic fibrosis and occurs in 10–15% of these cases. The condition is hereditary and transmitted by a recessive gene. In Western countries where the incidence of mucoviscidosis is in the region of 1 per 2,000 live births, meconium ileus is one of the commonest causes of intestinal obstruction in the newborn period, but in Africa and Asia it is relatively uncommon.

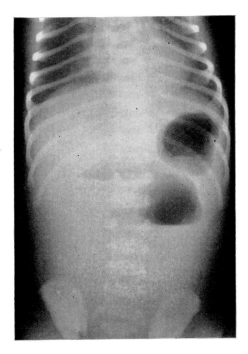

Figure 4.12b. Same case; erect film

The mucus-producing exocrine glands throughout the body become distended from retained viscid secretions. The pancreas is severely affected and the lack of pancreatic enzymes results in solidification of the meconium. Involvement of the liver may produce biliary cirrhosis, while pulmonary involvement leads to recurrent infections and ultimately fibrocystic disease. The effects on the intestinal tract range from temporary meconium retention with delayed but spontaneous evacuation of the meconium, to complete

79

obstruction. When obstruction occurs the distal ileum is narrowed and contains concretions of grey inspissated meconium pellets. Proximal to this the ileum is grossly distended by thick, tenacious, chewing-gum-like meconium due to the viscid, abnormal mucus. This dilated proximal loop of ileum may form the apex of a volvulus and small bowel atresia, secondary to intrauterine volvulus, may be found in some cases.

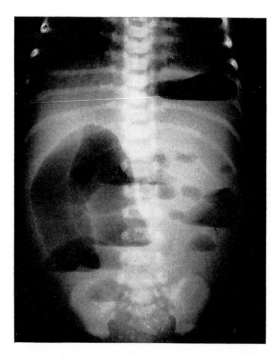

Figure 4.13. Erect film of ileal atresia; note how the distal ileal loop is more distended than the lower segments

Clinical features

Symptoms usually commence on the first day of life and consist of bile-stained vomiting and abdominal distension. The abdomen may have a doughy feel and it is sometimes possible to indent the bowel contents on pressure. Distended loops of bowel are frequently visible and sometimes peristalsis may be seen. Apart from an occasional mucus plug, very little meconium is passed per rectum. A family history is often elicited.

The diagnosis may be confirmed by finding an increased concentration of sodium chloride in the sweat. In infants this is facilitated by the pilocarpine iontophoresis sweat test. Concentrations of chloride of more than 60 mEq/l and sodium of more than 70 mEq/l are significant.

Radiological features

The plain films show multiple dilated loops of bowel which vary greatly in size (*Figure 4.14*). The erect film shows a lack of fluid levels,

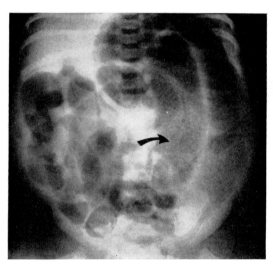

Figure 4.14. Meconium ileus; unequally distended bowel loops but no fluid levels is one of the significant features; the masses of speckled meconium (arrowed) are not specific for the condition

and although this is not an invariable feature, it should suggest the diagnosis. The sticky, viscid meconium prevents rapid movement of gas shadows during changes of posture so that fluid levels do not easily develop. Sometimes masses of meconium containing small bubbles of air may be visualized as coarse, granular, ground-glass shadows (*Figure 4.14*). It should be noted, however, that these masses are not pathognomonic of meconium ileus and may also be seen in other obstructions such as Hirschsprung's disease and ano-rectal malformations.

A contrast enema will reveal an unused microcolon. Characteristically the colon is minute and its diameter may be ribbon-like. If the terminal ileum is filled during the examination, meconium pellets may be visualized (*Figure 4.15*). Recently, Gastrografin enemas have been used in the treatment of the condition but the results of this form of treatment are not uniformly good and still await evaluation.

Meconium peritonitis

Meconium peritonitis results from intrauterine perforation of the

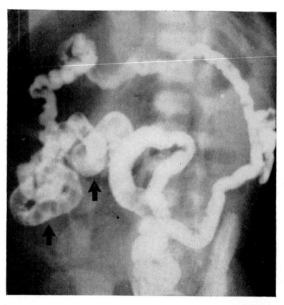

Figure 4.15. Contrast enema in a case of meconium ileus; note the extreme degree of 'microcolon'; the arrows show obstructing meconium in the terminal ileum

foetal gastrointestinal tract during the last six months of pregnancy. Sterile meconium escapes through the perforation into the peritoneal cavity producing a marked reaction with dense adhesions which usually calcify rapidly. Yellow-green nodules form on the bowel wall and the perforation may be sealed off so well that at birth there may not be any macroscopic evidence of the leak. However, if the perforation is still patent after birth and meconium still escapes into the peritoneal cavity, secondary septic peritonitis will develop. Very often a pseudocyst is formed by adjacent loops of intestine which tend to wall off the perforation. The wall of this pseudocyst is lined by a thick plaque of greenish-yellow material with areas of calcification.

The intrauterine perforation may be due to any obstructing lesion, e.g., atresia, meconium ileus, volvulus, Meckel's diverticulum, internal hernia, or bands. In such cases the causative lesion will be found at laparotomy. Not infrequently, however, no obvious cause for the perforation can be found. Such idiopathic perforations may be produced by localized areas of infarction due to minute emboli from the placenta.

Figure 4.16. Meconium peritonitis; small flakes of calcification (arrowed); the gas pattern shows some features of mechanical obstruction although there is free fluid in the abdomen

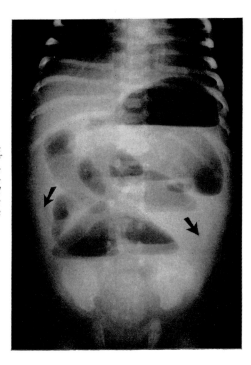

Clinical features

These babies are often hypothermic and in a poor condition due to septicaemia. The presenting features are those of intestinal obstruction, namely, vomiting, abdominal distension, and constipation.

The vomiting is bile-stained and may contain altered blood. Abdominal distension is obvious, and may be gross with a tight abdominal wall, distended veins, and respiratory embarrassment.

In infants in whom the meconium peritonitis is complicated by septic peritonitis, oedema and discolouration of the anterior abdominal wall may be evident.

Constipation is usually present and not infrequently altered blood may be passed per rectum or detected on rectal examination.

Radiological features

The diagnosis is usually obvious on the plain films of the abdomen. The calcification is intra-abdominal and extraluminal. It may form

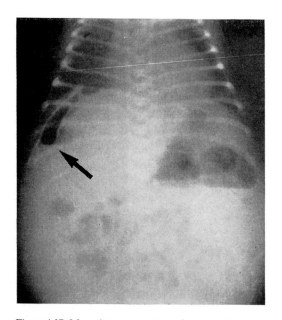

Figure 4.17. Meconium peritonitis; a plaque of calcification is forming a pseudocyst (arrow); free air in the peritoneal cavity is sealed off just above the head of the arrow

patchy amorphous masses or linear streaks. It may be difficult to see (*Figure 4.16*) but occasionally plaques will line a pseudocyst (*Figure 4.17*). In addition, distended loops of bowel with fluid levels due to the underlying intestinal obstruction are usually evident or may be present. Where the perforation is still patent, free air will be seen in the peritoneal cavity or trapped in a walled-off loculus or pseudocyst. The typical appearances of pneumoperitoneum are not usually seen in babies with meconium peritonitis because of the

84

presence of adhesions which obliterate most of the peritoneal cavity. Occasionally calcification may be seen in the scrotum when meconium has passed along a patent processus vaginalis into a hernial sac (*Figure 4.18*). It should be noted that a radiological diagnosis of meconium peritonitis can be made before birth if the peritoneal calcification in the foetus is dense enough to show up on x-rays of the mother's abdomen.

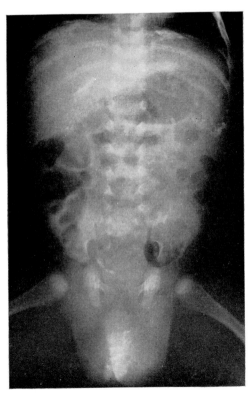

Figure 4.18. Meconium peritonitis with calcification extending in the scrotum

Functional obstruction

This term covers a group of conditions characterized by impaired intestinal motility without an obvious cause such as strangulating obstruction or peritonitis. We have noted the condition particularly in premature infants but it may occur in mature infants after recent abdominal surgery, sepsis, or therapy for tetanus neonatorum. In premature, debilitated infants it may be related to feeding the infant

85

on a formula containing an excessive concentration of powdered milk which tends to inspissate in the terminal ileum and colon. The water content of these inspissated pellets is lower (60%) than that of normal milk stools (80%) and we refer to the condition as the 'inspissated milk syndrome'.

Clinical features

The infant becomes obstructed after having initially passed meconium and later milk stools. The over-loaded intestines can often

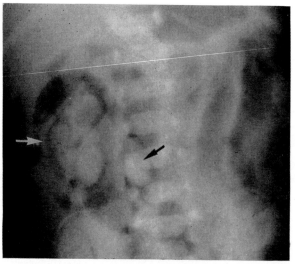

Figure 4.19a. Inspissated milk (caked curd), a cause of functional obstruction in a six-day-old premature. Fluid levels are not a feature and the opaque masses that are predominantly in small intestine have an air halo

be detected on palpation by a typical 'ropey feel' of the abdomen and may even be visible.

Radiological features

The plain films may show dense, amorphous, rounded or elongated intraluminal masses which are frequently surrounded by a halo of air (*Figure 4.19a*). Fluid levels are scarce. A Gastrografin contrast enema should be performed if the condition is suspected and the infant is not dehydrated. It may reveal rounded, filling defects due to the pellets of hardened curd (*Figure 4.19b*), and these are often evacuated at or soon after the examination.

Duplications

Duplications of the alimentary tract may occur at any level from the mouth to the anus. They have the same blood supply and share a common wall with the adjacent segments of the alimentary tract, but have a separate mucosal lining. They are invariably on the mesenteric side of the bowel and some may communicate with the alimentary tract. Their origin has not been adequately explained but they may represent persistence of vacuoles which are normally present during the solid stage of intestinal development.

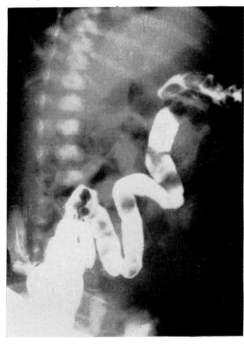

Figure 4.19b. Gastrografin enema in the same case, showing no colonic obstruction, but presence of dehydrated stool pellets. Rapid evacuation followed the enema with subsequent decompression

Two types of duplications are found:

(a) *Cystic* duplications are the common type and involve the small bowel, stomach, and duodenum. They are situated either in the mesentery or in the wall of the bowel and, since the secretions from the mucosal surface cannot escape, the cysts enlarge and usually present in the neonatal period with intestinal obstruction. This applies particularly to intramural duplication cysts commonly found in the terminal ileum. The mesenteric variety may present at a later stage with intestinal obstruction or as an intra-abdominal mass.

87

SMALL INTESTINE

(b) *Tubular* duplications usually communicate with the alimentary tract and often contain gastric mucosa. They occur most commonly in the colon but may involve the small bowel. Usually they present with massive haemorrhage due to peptic ulceration, or intestinal obstruction. A rare variant is the duplication which arises from the duodenum or jejunum and extends through the diaphragm into the

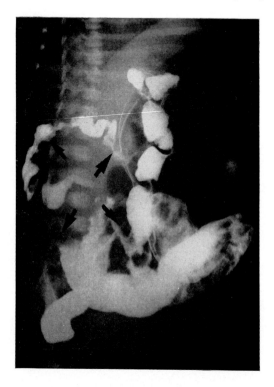

Figure 4.20. Barium enema, showing a rounded duplication cyst in the terminal ileum (arrows)

posterior mediastinum. This anomaly is commonly associated with hemivertebra in the cervical or upper dorsal regions (*Figure 1.9*), and forms part of the split notochord syndrome (see page 12).

Duplication cysts can be diagnosed on clinical grounds if a mass is felt, but often the condition is not suspected before laparotomy. A contrast enema may show a filling defect in the terminal ileum (*Figure 4.20*) or a contrast meal may show a large mass in the follow-through films. If the cyst contains gastric mucosa a diagnosis may be made by Technetium 99 scanning.

Miscellaneous

Small bowel intussusception and internal or external hernias are other rare causes of small intestinal obstruction in neonates. External hernias are obvious clinically, but the diagnosis of the other lesions is usually only made at surgery. A very long segment of aganglionosis involving the small bowel is another rare cause of small intestinal obstruction in the neonate and will be discussed further in Chapter 5.

5

The Large Intestine

After plain films the contrast enema is the most important examination in neonates with suspected intestinal obstruction. Because of the difficulty in distinguishing between large and small bowel on the plain films, the contrast enema is of particular importance in determining the site of the obstruction.

Technique of contrast enema

It is most important to have a safe standard technique and the following routine covers the important points.

(a) *Handling the infant:* sick infants must be handled with great gentleness and care. They are very sensitive to temperature changes and must not be kept out of incubators for prolonged periods. During the examination the baby should be kept covered and if the diagnosis is not evident on fluoroscopy, the infant must be returned to the incubator while waiting for the films to be developed.

(b) *Contrast media:* a 30% W/V solution of barium is an excellent, cheap, and safe contrast medium. If, during the examination, a diagnosis of meconium plug or meconium ileus is made, the barium should be siphoned off and Gastrografin injected (this is a hypertonic solution and should not be used if the infant is clinically dehydrated).

(c) *Technique of examination:* a small pile of gauze swabs is placed under the infant. These are easily slipped out and replaced when barium leakage occurs. A 50 ml syringe is used to inject barium through a soft rubber 8–10 French catheter. Inflatable, balloon-type catheters should never be used in neonates because of the danger of rupturing the bowel at the rectosigmoid junction. Manual injection gives good control of the barium flow and a second syringe, already filled, is kept at hand to avoid delay in continuity if more barium should be required.

90

With the infant in the lateral position, a moist but unlubricated catheter is inserted into the anus and advanced 2 to 4 cm. It should lie in the distal rectum above the puborectalis sling. A few millilitres are initially injected to visualize the condition of the rectum and to note the presence of any low contracted area. The tube is then advanced a further 2 cm and the child turned on to its back with the legs firmly extended. To prevent expulsion of the enema tube an assistant should gently squeeze the buttocks together with his fingers whilst the radiation field is coned down to exclude his hands. If there is still difficulty in getting the infant to retain the barium, it may be better to carry out the examination with the baby in the prone position when its buttocks can be controlled more effectively and the assistant's hands kept out of the radiation field. (Using this technique the radiation to the unprotected hand is negligible—after three minutes fluoroscopy we have monitored only 0·006 rad. Radiologists should check their own units and if required rotate the assisting staff.) Adhesive tape is commonly used, but it is better dispensed with as it is often ineffective and attention to this detail distracts attention from the important early filling changes.

The infant's sigmoid colon is normally redundant and ascends well out of the pelvis. While it is being filled the radiologist should pause to consider the diagnosis of Hirschsprung's disease, as too rapid filling may over-distend the aganglionic segment. The bowel should be visualized and appropriate films taken in the lateral, oblique, and AP positions. Some slight rotation of the infant may be necessary to visualize the splenic flexure and the location of the transverse colon and, finally, the position of the caecum should be carefully studied when abnormalities of rotation are in question.

The following abnormalities may be demonstrated during the examination.

Colon pathology
  (a) Hirschsprung's disease
  (b) Necrotizing enterocolitis
  (c) Anomalies of rotation and midgut volvulus
  (d) Colonic atresia or stenosis
  (e) Meconium plug syndrome
  (f) Intussusception

Small bowel pathology
  (a) Small bowel atresia
  (b) Meconium ileus

(c) Functional obstruction
(d) Duplication cysts of the terminal ileum

HIRSCHSPRUNG'S DISEASE

In recent years there has been a tendency to refer to Hirschsprung's disease as aganglionosis, or congenital aganglionic megacolon or, more correctly, congenital intestinal aganglionosis, but the eponym 'Hirschsprung's disease' has become so well established that it will probably stay. Because of the difficulties in making a diagnosis by contrast enema the diagnostic features will be considered in some detail.

Aetiology and pathogenesis

The essential lesion is congenital absence of ganglia in the sub-mucosal and intermuscular myenteric plexuses of the distal part of the bowel. Their place is taken by clusters of enlarged, unmedullated nerve fibres. The aganglionosis commences at the lower end of the rectum and extends proximally for a variable distance. In about 80% of cases the anomaly does not extend beyond the sigmoid (short segment), while in the remainder it extends proximally to involve variable lengths of the colon and may even involve the terminal ileum (long segment). Very rarely it involves the whole of the small as well as the large bowel. The aganglionic segment remains unexpanded and the proximal colon becomes distended and hypertrophied. The severity of symptoms does not depend entirely on the length of the aganglionic segment.

The great rarity of the anomaly in premature infants suggests that the ganglia might be destroyed late in foetal life. The natural distribution of aganglionosis, the rarity of 'skip lesions' and the absence of aganglionosis in atresias and stenoses, renders a vascular cause unlikely, and experimentally, temporary ischaemia to a segment of colon has failed to produce aganglionosis.

Considerable evidence obtained from family studies as well as from animal experimentation has now accumulated to incriminate genetic factors. The experimental work of Yntema and Hammond (1954) suggests that Hirschsprung's disease is due to a disturbance in the migration of cells from the craniocervical portion of the embryonic neural tube to the gut.

The embryological studies of Okomoto and Ueda have further substantiated the concept that aganglionosis is a developmental anomaly in which transcaudal migration of neuroblasts into the

92

alimentary tract has been arrested at varying stages before the twelfth week of gestation. The rectosigmoid, being the most distal part, is the most common site to be involved, but with earlier arrest of migration the segment of aganglionosis will be correspondingly longer.

Several workers have studied the response to drugs in cases of Hirschsprung's disease. Strips of muscle from the aganglionic segment are less sensitive to acetylcholine than in normal controls. Kamijo *et al.* (1953) found an increase of specific and nonspecific cholinesterase activity in the aganglionic bowel and, by histochemical studies, showed that this finding was closely associated with the abnormal nerve fibres. Ehrenpreis (1952) has shown that substance P (a biologically active polypeptide found in nerve tissue), which stimulates smooth muscle activity, is greatly reduced in the aganglionic segment and increased in the hypertrophied proximal colon. Wright and Shepherd found that aganglionic muscle responds normally to adrenaline but is contracted by nicotine, and suggest that an adrenergic-inhibiting system is absent or functionally subnormal. Further histochemical studies have shown that adrenergic nerve fibres to normal intestines are distributed mainly to the intramural plexuses where they make synaptic contacts with the parasympathetic ganglion cells. In Hirschsprung's disease these adrenergic synapses are lacking in the aganglionic segment.

Further interesting work has been done by Ehrenpreis and his group (1968) on the pathophysiology of the condition. By histochemical flourescent studies they showed that the mediation not only of parasympathetic but also of sympathetic influences to the aganglionic bowel is interrupted. This functional denervation promotes spastic contraction which is the main characteristic of the distal aganglionic segment in Hirschsprung's disease. Further studies along these lines are clearly indicated and may be rewarding.

Clinical features

With increasing awareness of the early symptomatology of Hirschsprung's disease it is now realized that the child with 'classical' abdominal distension, severe constipation, stunted growth, and wasted limbs is the survivor of a relatively minor form of the disease. More often it causes more urgent symptoms (obstruction or diarrhoea) in the neonate or during early infancy and, if untreated, at least 50% will succumb during the first year of life. With a high index of suspicion the diagnosis can be made during the first days or weeks of life. Paediatricians are aware of this and during the past five years over 70% (38 cases, sex ratio 3 M:1 F) of new cases of Hirschsprung's disease admitted to the Red Cross War Memorial Children's Hospital, Cape Town, have been neonates. These have all had x-ray appearances that were diagnostic or indicated the need for biopsy.

Usually the infants are well at birth, but within a few days they become distended, often vomit and the passage of meconium is

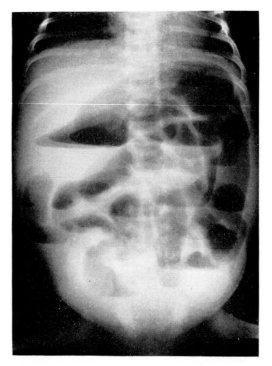

Figure 5.1. Hirschsprung's disease (short segment); plain film showing low small bowel obstruction

delayed. The constipation is sometimes relieved spontaneously or, more often, after digital examination of the rectum.

The acute episode, which may be mild and transient or severe and life-threatening, represents the initial 'decompensation period'. Failure to recognize the lesion at this stage may be responsible for a disastrous outcome in the form of acute obstruction and enterocolitis, or prolonged suffering depending upon the subsequent progress, which may conform to any of the following patterns:

Group I: acute obstruction persists until death or relief by colostomy (or ileostomy in total colonic aganglionosis).

Group II: recurrent obstructive episodes occur, necessitating early colostomy.

Group III: recurrent obstructive episodes occur but respond well to washouts.

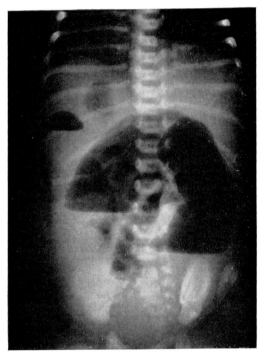

Figure 5.2. Hirschsprung's disease (short segment); plain film showing obstruction with dilated sigmoid loop

Group IV: the 'compensated' case. Mild obstructive symptoms occur but tend to settle, although constipation is often a problem. Over a period of a year or so the 'classical' clinical picture may develop.

Group V: attacks of enterocolitis occur and these are lethal in 25–50% of affected infants.

Enterocolitis, the dreaded complication, is said to occur in 50% of infants suffering from aganglionosis. It is characterized by severe prostration, massive abdominal distension despite enemas, foul watery diarrhoea, and sometimes vomiting. Dehydration develops out of all proportion to the external losses and the infant may die within 24 hours. Those who recover are prone to further attacks.

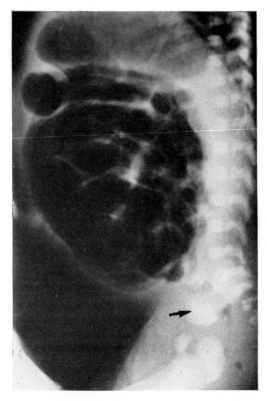

Figure 5.3. Hirschsprung's disease (short segment); lateral inverted film showing 'egg on end' appearance with a small amount of gas in the affected rectosigmoid region

Enterocolitis can be avoided by the timely performance of a proximal colostomy.

Manometric studies
Recently Lawson and Nixon (1967) and Tobon *et al.* (1968) have shown that manometric studies of the anal canal and the rectum are of

value in the diagnosis of Hirschsprung's disease. In normal subjects distension of the rectum produces relaxation of the internal sphincter and contraction of the external sphincter, whereas in patients with Hirschsprung's disease there is contraction of the internal sphincter.

Rectal biopsy
    Confirmation of the diagnosis by histological examination is neces-

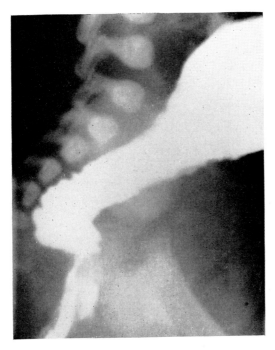

*Figure 5.4. Typical short segment Hirschsprung's disease;
note the low insertion of the catheter during the early stages
of the injection; the transition zone is well demonstrated*

sary before definitive treatment is carried out. The biopsy of the rectal wall must be taken at least 2 cm from the mucocutaneous junction because below this point ganglion cells are often scanty or absent in normal subjects. Of the several methods used to obtain the biopsy specimen, the technique described by Swenson and Fisher (1959) and MacMahon *et al.* (1963) has been widely adopted but suction biopsy may prove to be an improvement on this.

The timing of the rectal biopsy is important. In older infants and children it should be done as soon as the diagnosis is suspected. When the definitive resection of the aganglionic segment is performed soon after the biopsy, some surrounding inflammatory reaction at the biopsy site is always found, and there is a tendency for the biopsy scar to split during mobilization of the rectum. It is, therefore,

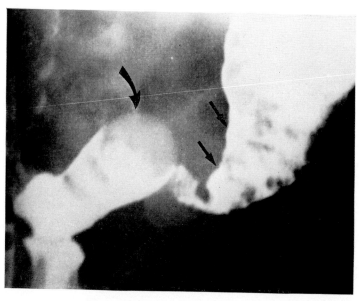

Figure 5.5. Short segment Hirschsprung's disease; the rectal region (curved arrow) is dilated by impacted faeces; the transition zone (arrows) shows some rippling or fine notching of its contour margins

preferable to obtain a frozen section report at the time of the biopsy and to proceed with the resection immediately, or better still, to postpone resection for several weeks to allow adequate healing of the biopsy site.

In neonates presenting with acute obstruction which cannot be relieved by washouts, an immediate colostomy sited proximal to the transitional zone is required. In such cases biopsies must be taken at the site for frozen section examination to ensure that ganglia are, in fact, present. In addition, if the condition of the infant permits, biopsies should be taken of the distal collapsed bowel to confirm the diagnosis of Hirschsprung's disease.

In infants in whom the obstructive episode has been relieved by washouts and the diagnosis has been confirmed radiologically, it may be tempting to omit the rectal biopsy because the procedure is difficult in small infants. However, mistakes have been made and

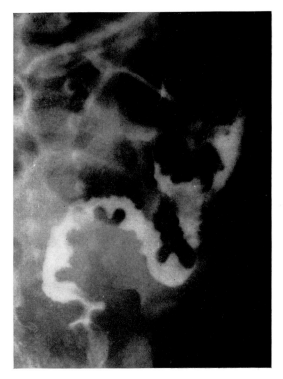

Figure 5.6. Typical appearances of sigmoid Hirschsprung's disease, this is an 'early' delayed film after minimal filling

such chances cannot be taken before embarking on surgical treatment.

Radiological diagnosis

Plain films

Hirschsprung's disease should be suspected in every infant who presents with clinical evidence of obstruction and multiple fluid levels on the plain x-ray. The gas distribution usually shows low bowel obstruction (*Figure 5.1*) and in the common, short segment cases the distended loop of sigmoid colon may be seen on the AP film (*Figure 5.2*). This appearance should not be confused with that of sigmoid volvulus which, in adults, is somewhat similar. Occasionally, the inverted lateral film may show the narrowed segment outlined

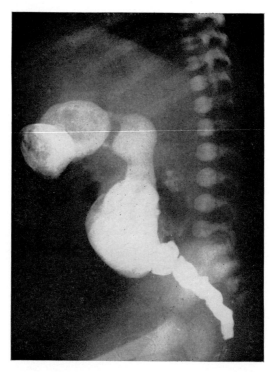

Figure 5.7. 'Late' delayed film showing the narrowed rectosigmoid area well visualized in this lateral projection

with air and the distended abdomen has an 'egg on end' appearance (*Figure 5.3*) Linear strips of intramural air are uncommon but may occur if there has been gross overdistension.

Contrast enema

The radiologist conducting the examination must examine the sigmoid colon slowly and carefully. The examination is best performed with a 30% W/V barium suspension, preferably before washouts are given. Under these conditions the danger of water intoxication is minimized. The basic diagnostic points are the demonstration of a relatively narrowed area, a transition zone which cones up into a dilated colon, and retention of barium in a 'late' delayed (12–24 hour) film. This, however, over-simplifies the problem in neonates, because the changes outlined may take up to two weeks to be recog-

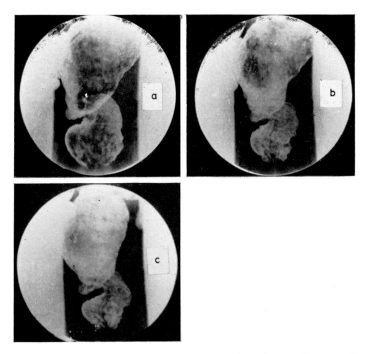

Figure 5.8. Serial 70 mm films in a 3 year old infant showing the purposeless churning contractions of the aganglionic area

nizable, particularly if washouts have been given to relieve the condition, or the aganglionic segment is long.

Short-segment aganglionosis: The following features may be noted on barium enema.

(a) Relative narrowing of the aganglionic segment (*Figures 5.4 and 5.5*). This can easily be missed in the early part of the examination if too rapid filling causes over-distension. While injecting the barium, the radiologist should pause to assess the condition of the sigmoid colon as soon as it has filled. The narrowing of the aganglionic segment is only relative and portions of the colon or rectum may be dilated by impacted faecal material (*Figure 5.5*).

(b) The transition zone, i.e., a cone-shaped area where the narrow, distal bowel widens out to join the proximal dilated bowel may also be missed if filling is too rapid, which is liable to occur when a water-

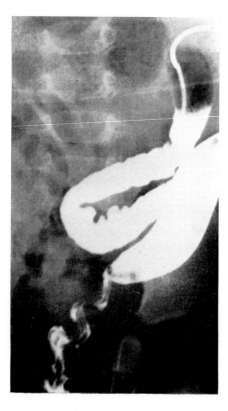

Figure 5.9. Gastrografin loopogram on an infant admitted with a transverse colostomy performed elsewhere; this examination showed the diagnosis and enabled the biopsy to be taken at the correct transition zone

soluble contrast medium is used instead of barium. The commencement of the dilated area is the important zone to be watched. Sometimes the colon margin in this region has a finely notched appearance (*Figure 5.5*).

(c) A dilated area above the narrowed area (*Figure 5.6*). This is the classical megacolon of the older child. It is not gross in neonates and may take some weeks to develop fully. This feature is particularly difficult to assess when relieving washouts have been previously given.

(d) Retention of barium in a 'late' delayed 12–24 hour lateral film (*Figure 5.7*). We have found this a most valuable film for confirming a suspected diagnosis of Hirschsprung's disease. A lateral film shows the narrowed segment best with the barium uniformly distributed within it. The aganglionic segment will frequently appear to be in a spastic state. We have observed spastic contractions, which are nonpropulsive, in the affected segment of older children (*Figure*

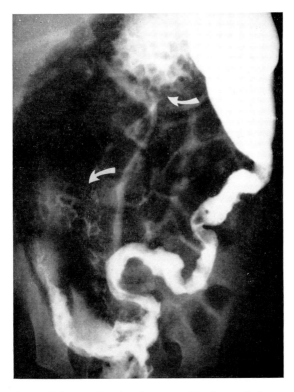

Figure 5.10. A medium length segment Hirschsprung's disease in an 'early' delayed film; the arrows point to the cobblestone mucosal appearance of enterocolitis

5.8), but do not advise post-enema fluoroscopy to observe this phenomenon in neonates. The main problem in regard to delayed films is that the infant may be so ill that surgery or relieving rectal washouts may be necessary soon after the initial examination. Superadded enterocolitis, which causes rapid evacuation of barium,

103

also compromises the value of delayed films. However, with careful examination it is usually possible to diagnose the common type of short segment Hirschsprung's disease on the first examination. Nevertheless, there should be no hesitation in repeating the examination if there is any radiological or clinical doubt. The second examination is usually easier and the radiologist can be more confident of his findings. The important feature to look for is the transition from relatively narrow to dilated colon. We terminate the examination if

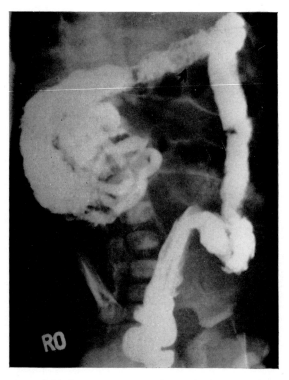

Figure 5.11. Long segment Hirschsprung's disease involving entire colon and terminal ileum; enterocolitis is also present (arrow)

dilation is found, the relative changes will then be better appreciated. They are often best seen a few minutes after the catheter has been removed, therefore an 'early' delayed film should always be taken after the examination has terminated (*Figure 5.6*).

(e) Cases may be referred in which a colostomy has been performed to relieve the obstruction without a diagnosis being made. A distal loopogram in these cases gives diagnostic information and shows the site at which biopsy should be taken (*Figure 5.9*).

Long-segment Hirschsprung's disease: In these cases the diagnosis by barium enema can be extremely difficult during the first few days

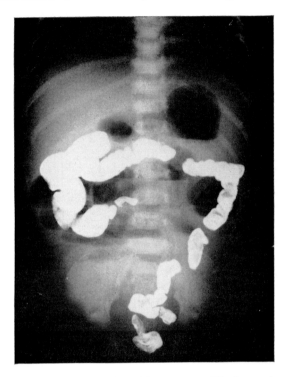

Figure 5.12. Delayed film of long segment Hirschsprung's disease involving entire colon; this film was taken on admission to this hospital, three days after a barium enema had been performed elsewhere

of life. The colon proximal to the aganglionic segment has not had time to become a recognizable dilated reservoir and these cases, in particular, may require a second examination (*Figure 5.10*). The whole colon is involved in 5% of cases and, rarely, the distal ileum is also affected (*Figure 5.11*). Such cases are not easy to diagnose radiologically. The appearance of the colon is variable; it may be distended by faecal material or relatively narrowed or shortened or apparently normal. We do not advise over-filling of the terminal

105

ileum because of the risk of complete small bowel reflux with vomiting and aspiration pneumonia.

Delayed films will show retention of barium throughout the colon and there may be a 'minicolon' appearance because of relative shortening (*Figure 5.12*). However, this 'spastic shortening', particularly of the sigmoid colon, although often present in delayed films, is not a reliable sign during the filling stage of the examination.

Summary of x-ray findings

Plain films: if taken during acute attacks these films will show evidence of intestinal obstruction with distended loops of bowel and air/fluid levels. The lateral inverted film may have an 'egg-on-end' appearance and sometimes narrowing of the rectal gas shadow may be detected.

Barium enema:

(a) As the barium flows through the anal canal to fill the rectum and pelvic colon, the diagnostic pattern, namely narrowed distal bowel followed by a cone-shaped transitional area followed by dilated bowel, will be revealed. This will always be present on careful examination but the pattern becomes less apparent in long-segment aganglionosis.

(b) When the suspected area of transition has been filled no more barium should be injected and the catheter withdrawn. The area should then be carefully rescreened and the examination not concluded till a further film has been taken. The narrow aganglionic area is often best seen in an AP or lateral 'early' delayed film. A 'late' delayed film (12–24 hour) will show barium retention and may also show the narrowed area to advantage.

(c) Enterocolitis causes mucosal changes and spastic areas which may render the diagnosis extremely difficult (*Figure 5.14*).

(d) The presence of a meconium plug must always arouse suspicion of Hirschsprung's disease.

ENTEROCOLITIS

The aetiology of this condition remains obscure, but in the 'necrotizing' enterocolitis of prematures it appears to be initially an aseptic condition. The high incidence of prematurity (about 80%) and abnormal pregnancies in the necrotizing variety suggests that in these cases it may be the effect of hypoxia activating a defence mechanism, whereby the blood is shunted from the mesenteric vessels to more vital areas. This results in selective intestinal ischaemia which causes mucosal necrosis and allows gas and bacteria to enter the submucosa.

The important radiological features on the plain films are gaseous distension of the bowel, often with excessive air fluid levels and intramural gas (*see* p. 40 and *Figures 2.3, 2.4* and *2.5*). A pneumoperitoneum (*Figures 2.6* and *2.7*) indicates a perforation, while gas in the portal veins (*Figure 2.9*) indicates a probable fatal outcome. The thin translucent lines of portal venous gas may be transient and are sometimes best seen in a lateral view. All these cases require constant

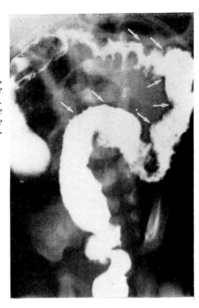

Figure 5.13. Necrotizing enterocolitis, the arrows point to the gas in the bowel wall (same case as Figure 2.4). We do not advise enemas in these cases. It was performed with extreme caution, because of a clinical suspicion of intussusception

clinical and radiological surveillance and immediate surgery is indicated if the condition of the infant deteriorates or the radiographs show a pneumoperitoneum. Later complications include stricture and internal fistula formation. Barium enema will seldom be required to make the diagnosis and due to the risk of perforation it is not advised. A shaggy outline or fine spicules protruding beyond the contour of the bowel are caused by the mucosal ulceration (*Figure 5.13*). A thumbprinting or cobblestone appearance is caused by mucosal oedema. The colon is usually empty and it is important to note that alterations in calibre with pseudo-transitional areas may resemble the 'coning' of Hirschsprung's disease and lead to an erroneous diagnosis. In the enterocolitis of Hirschsprung's disease (*see* p. 96), we have not yet definitely noted the presence of intramural gas. This sign is difficult to evaluate in overdistended bowel,

107

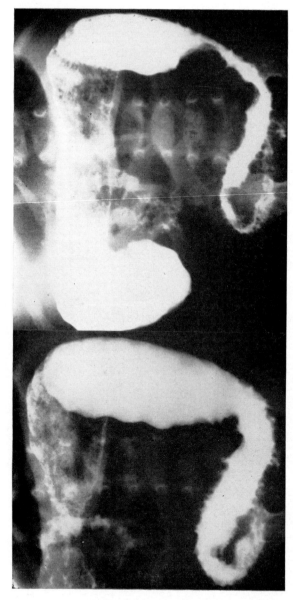

Figure 5.14. Severe enterocolitis in a two-week-old Hirschsprung's disease. Note the calibre changes in the same examination and the spicules produced by ulceration of the lower colon; this case initially presented as a meconium plug

but its uncommon appearance in Hirschsprung's disease may result from overdistension. A barium enema may give similar appearances with spastic areas and mucosal oedema (*Figure 5.14*). It should be noted that the necrotising variety of enterocolitis occurs predominantly in prematures and is prone to intramural gas, whereas Hirschsprung's disease is rare in prematures and the complicating enterocolitis is not prone to intramural gas. It is likely that these two types of enterocolitis have a different basic aetiology.

ABNORMALITIES OF ROTATION

When atresias of the small bowel are associated with rotational anomalies the diagnosis of the malrotation can usually be made on

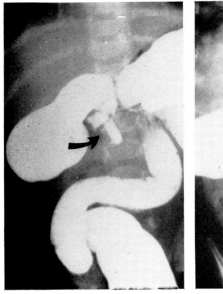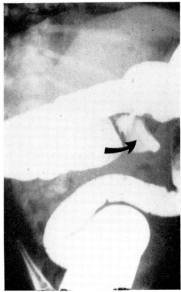

Figure 5.15. Barium enema on a case of malrotation, the arrow points to the caecum and appendix which are situated high in the midline (AP and lateral oblique views)

barium enema. In such cases the position of the unused microcolon and caecum is self evident.

In the typical Ladd's syndrome where the caecum is situated in the subhepatic or midabdominal position, a definite diagnosis can also be made on barium enema (*Figure 5.15*). Conversely, if malrotation is suspected and the barium enema reveals a normally situated

109

caecum, such a diagnosis can be ruled out. On the other hand, minor variations in the height of the caecum may be very difficult to assess. In such cases it is useful to note whether there is any sudden deviation downwards of the mid-transverse colon while the barium is being injected. If this should be seen, additional barium must be injected very slowly to facilitate assessment of the position of the

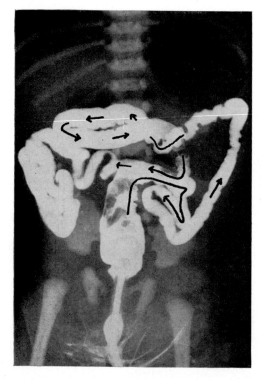

Figure 5.16. Microcolon in a case of jejunal atresia; the colon followed a complicated course of malrotation

proximal colon before over filling renders evaluation impossible (*Figure 5.16*). When malrotation is complicated by midgut volvulus, the caecum and right colon may form part of the volvulus, in which case the barium may not pass beyond the right transverse colon.

COLONIC ATRESIA AND STENOSIS

In colonic atresia the barium enema will reveal an unused microcolon up to the point of occlusion. The condition may be associated with more proximal small bowel atresias which may be detected on plain films. In colonic stenosis the enema will demonstrate a persistent narrowing with a variable degree of dilatation of the more proximal colon (*Figure 5.17*).

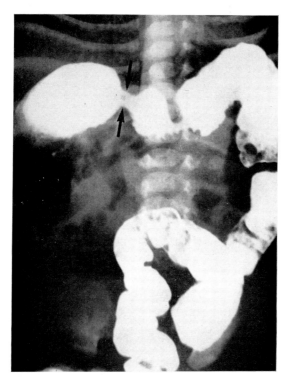

Figure 5.17. Stenosis of the colon (arrowed), narrowing remained persistent during the barium enema

MECONIUM PLUG

This is a relatively benign form of low intestinal obstruction which usually presents in the first few days of life. The aetiology of the condition is obscure and it is not associated with cystic fibrosis. The meconium forms a long, thick, snake-like plug which obstructs the colon.

The plain films will show fluid levels indicating distal intestinal obstruction, and there may be considerable dilatation of the colon, best seen on the lateral films. The contrast enema will reveal the plug

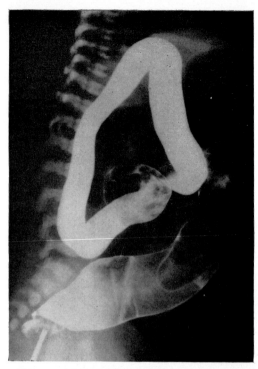

Figure 5.18a. Meconium plug demonstrated by Gastro-grafin enema

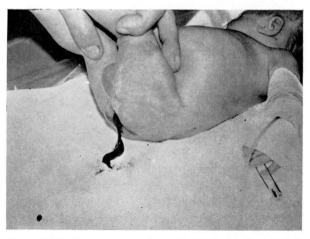

Figure 5.18b. Same case; on flexing the thighs at the end of the examination part of the meconium plug was extruded

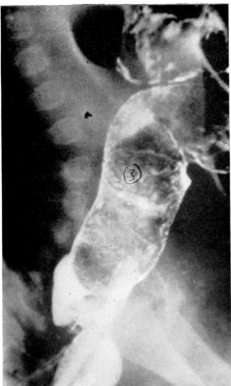

Figure 5.19. Intussusception in the rectum, initially the intussusception almost prevented the insertion of the catheter into the rectum

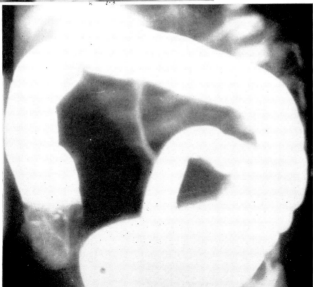

Figure 5.20. Intussusception at the hepatic flexure in a month old infant

as a translucent filling defect surrounded by opaque material. Barium will sometimes stream around the plug to give a double contrast appearance, with the contrast-lined colonic walls showing up against the negative filling defect of the plug (*Figure 5.18a*).

When a diagnosis of meconium plug is made on fluoroscopy, the contrast medium should be changed to Gastrografin which will assist in evacuation of the plug. After 50 ml of Gastrografin have been injected, the infant's hips should be gently hyperflexed to compress the abdomen. With this manoeuvre the Gastrografin will squirt out together with part of the plug (*Figure 5.18b*). The plug may be surprisingly long and the effect of its evacuation is similar to that of removing a bung from a barrel.

A number of cases of meconium plug have been associated with Hirschsprung's disease and we have found this association particularly common with extensive plugs (three in our last five cases). It is, therefore, important to repeat the contrast enema at a later stage before regarding the plug as the sole cause of the obstruction.

INTUSSUSCEPTION

This condition is more frequent in older children, being most common in males, from the sixth to twenty-fourth month. It may, however, occur in the first six weeks of life when the ileocaecal or ileocolic varieties are usually encountered, although the sigmoid type may sometimes occur. Bloodstained mucus is frequently passed and the infant usually cries out during attacks of abdominal colic. An abdominal mass may be palpable and in the sigmoid variety, in particular, the intussusception may present at the anus and resemble rectal prolapse (*Figure 5.19*).

In the neonate the plain films, apart from indicating some obstruction, are not usually diagnostic. On barium enema the diagnosis is not difficult because the head of the retrograde column of barium ends abruptly in a lobster-claw-like deformity (*Figure 5.20*). Sometimes the barium may penetrate between the layers of the intussusception to give a watchspring appearance. If the technique of neonatal examination described by us is adopted, we do not advise attempts at complete reduction of the intussusception by barium enema.

6

Anorectal Malformations

Malformations of the rectum and anus are among the commonest serious congenital abnormalities encountered. The incidence in Cape Town is approximately 1 in 1,800 births and our remarks are based on our experience with 287 infants suffering from anorectal malformations treated from 1954 through 1969. It is a sad, but true fact, that these malformations are generally more poorly understood and more badly handled than any other congenital anomaly in the newborn.

The malformations include a wide spectrum of defects ranging from minor aberrations of the anus to most complex and serious anomalies of rectum and anus, often associated with other major congenital abnormalities.

A detailed description of the various anomalies is unnecessary and may be found elsewhere. Suffice it to say that the crucial factor is the relationship of the terminal bowel to the levator ani muscle, and in particular, to the puborectalis component of this muscle. At the Paediatric Surgical Congress held at the Royal Children's Hospital in Melbourne in 1970 it was agreed that the classification set out below might be acceptable, but it must be emphasized that it is a compromise and modification of many classifications and ideas previously published.

A High or Supralevator Anomalies
  (where the bowel ends above the pelvic floor)
  1 *Anorectal Agenesis*
    (a) Without fistula
    (b) With fistula—Males: Rectovesical
                            Recto-urethral
              Females: Rectovesical
                        Rectocloacal
                        Rectovaginal (high)

2 *Rectal Atresia*
(anal canal present)

B Intermediate Anomalies
(where the bowel is embraced by the puborectalis muscle)

1 *Anal Agenesis*
(a) Without fistula
(b) With fistula—Males: Rectobulbar
Females: Rectovaginal (low)
Rectovestibular

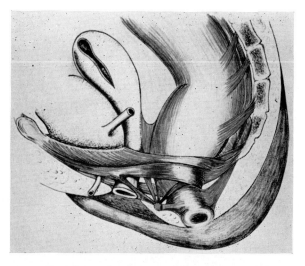

Figure 6.1. Puborectalis sling embracing rectum and urethra to form the muscle floor of the pelvis and dividing high from low lesions

2 *Anorectal Senosis*
(anal canal present)

C Low or Translevator Anomalies
(where bowel ends below the pelvic floor)

1 *At normal anal site*
(a) Covered anus
(b) Anal stenosis
2 *At perineal site*
(a) Anocutaneous fistula
(b) Anterior perineal anus

3 *At vulvar site*
  (a) Vulvar anus
  (b) Anovulval fistula
  (c) Anovestibular fistula

D   **Miscellaneous**
  (uncommon abnormalities not belonging to the above groups)

In the diagnosis and management of any particular case, it is most important to determine the relationship of the terminal bowel

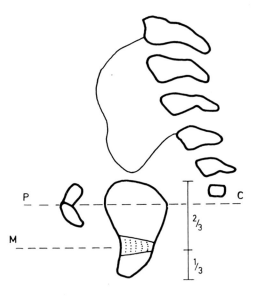

Figure 6.2. 'M' point at the junction of upper two-thirds and lower third of bony ischium; it lies below the PC line and marks the position of puborectalis more accurately. It is not a rigid point and with gross over-distension it may descend down to lower ischium but not beyond

to the puborectalis. This may be possible from the clinical presentation alone but often radiological assessment is required for a diagnosis. The latter is based primarily on the position of the gas in the terminal bowel as seen on lateral films of the inverted baby, but contrast studies are not infrequently necessary for accuracy. The differentiation between high and low anomalies used to be determined by the distance of the gas from a skin marker at the anal site—but this method is hopelessly inaccurate. Since 1953 the so-called pubococcygeal line described by Douglas Stephens (1971) has been used as the dividing line between high and low anomalies. However, it is obvious from *Figure 6.1* that a line drawn from the pubic bone to the sacrococcygeal junction is well above the levator sling. We, therefore, utilize the ischium as the bony landmark indicative of the level of the levator sling. Loopograms have shown that the junction of the upper two thirds and lower third of the ischium is at the level of the pelvic floor and we have designated this point on the bone as the 'M' (muscle) point (*Figure 6.2*). The puborectalis may contract or bulge slightly within the area of the 'M' point, but utilizing this landmark we have differentiated without error our last fifty cases into high and low abnormalities. We now use the 'M' point rather than the pubococcygeal line because the latter does not accurately delineate the site of puborectalis and may be difficult to define—frequently the lower sacral segments are absent and the pubic rami, which form a boomerang-shaped shadow, are difficult to visualize.

RADIOLOGICAL METHODS OF EXAMINATION

The methods used to study these cases are:

(a) Plain films: Routine scout films with pelvic inverted lateral film (*Figures 6.5a, 6.6a, 6.7a, 6.11, 6.14a*)

(b) Loopograms: Contrast medium injected into the distal loop of a colostomy, i.e., into a defunctioning colostomy before definitive surgery (*Figures 6.5b, 6.5c, 6.6b, 6.7b, 6.7c, 6.8, 6.10, 6.12, 6.13*)

(c) Fistulograms: (*Figures 6.9, 6.15, 6.16*)

(d) Urogenital examinations

Plain films

There has been a recent tendency to decry the usefulness of plain films but properly taken they may provide the following useful information:

(a) The level of the lesion

(b) The presence of gas in the bladder indicating a high lesion

(c) The presence of complications such as hydrocolpos

(d) Associated sacral or vertebral anomalies.

The assessment of the films must be correlated with prior knowledge of the infant's sex, the clinical appearance of the perineum, the direction of a fistulous track, and the presence of meconium in the urine. In this assessment the lateral inverted film can differentiate accurately between high and blind low lesions. However, when there is a patent vaginal or perineal fistula gas will escape and not be trapped in the pelvis, thus rendering the plain films worthless. These fistulae are usually found in girls in whom an accurate clinical diagnosis can be made.

For adequate visualization of the ischial bones and accurate assessment of the relation of the gas shadow to the 'M' point, the following technique should be used:

(a) The infant should be at least twelve hours old to ensure that gas has reached the rectal region.

(b) The x-ray tube must be centred in a true lateral position on the buttock region (*Figure 6.3*). It is a common error to take the

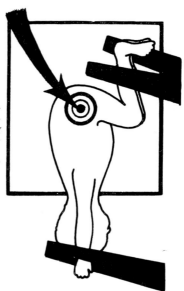

Figure 6.3. Position of inverted infant for x-ray target zone for the ischium is the midbuttock area, note flexed thighs and extended arms. The radiologist must personally be involved in checking adequate inversion if accurate results are to be obtained

inverted film centred around the middle of the abdomen when the important bony points are displaced to a far corner of the film.

(c) The thighs should be well flexed to clear the femora from most of the ischium (*Figure 6.4*).

(d) The arms should be extended around the back of the head to splint the body and prevent excessive movement. It is best to use two pairs of hands to suspend the infant.

(e) The infant should be held in the inverted position for at least seven minutes to allow air to enter the most distal portion of the

119

rectum. If too short a time has been allowed and the x-ray findings are doubtful, the film should be repeated.

It is an advantage for the child to cry because the respiratory movements force the air in the bowel down to the termination of the blind end. We have found that with the above technique impacted meconium does not prevent gas from reaching the end of the bowel.

Loopograms

High lesions are initially treated by colostomy and, at a later convenient time, the level and nature of the lesion can, therefore, be

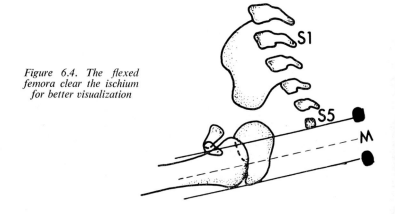

Figure 6.4. The flexed femora clear the ischium for better visualization

studied further by injecting contrast material down the distal loop. This examination is performed under fluoroscopic control by using a water soluble contrast material and a French 5 Foley-type catheter which is inserted into the colostomy opening. A transverse colostomy requires 20–40 ml contrast material. When a sigmoid colostomy has been performed much less is injected as the distal colonic loop is very short and great caution must be exercised to avoid excessive pressure which may rupture the bowel. Water soluble contrast media and not barium should be used in all cases and if the bladder should fill, vesico-ureteric reflux may also be seen.

As the sigmoid colon begins to fill the infant must be turned into the lateral position to permit adequate examination of the rectal region. After the rectum has been expanded the injection should be interrupted because the compressing effect of crying movements tends to fill the fistulous tract more easily than an increase in the

120

injection pressure does (*Figures 6.5b, 6.5c*). Most high lesions with fistulae occur in males in whom the fistulae commonly enter the mid-prostatic urethra. These fistulae may be very narrow and the bladder neck is often elongated and kinked backwards at the site of the fistula (*Figure 6.6b*). Indeed, it is because of the narrowness of the fistula that this method of demonstrating it is preferred to retrograde micturition cysto-urethrography.

Fistulograms

The examination is performed by passing a French 5 plastic feeding tube into the fistula and injecting water soluble contrast medium.

If the anatomy of a lesion is obvious from perineal inspection fistulograms are usually unnecessary. We find them most useful in females with low anomalies associated with fistulae in the perineum or vulva. Most vaginal fistulae are associated with supralevator lesions, but it is not always easy to decide if the fistula is situated in the lower vagina or in the vestibular–vulvar area. The fistulogram may also differentiate intermediate lesions, such as anal agenesis with rectovestibular fistula from low lesions, such as anovulvar or vestibular fistulae.

Fistulae opening into a urogenital sinus can also be demonstrated by this method; in these cases it is better to insert a French 5 Foley catheter inflated with 2 cc of air into the cloacal opening and to inject the contrast material through the catheter. This method is more satisfactory than blunt syringe flushing techniques.

HIGH OR SUPRALEVATOR ANOMALIES

These account for 40% of our cases. They are always serious because:

(a) Despite the usual presence of a fistulous opening there is almost always severe obstruction.

(b) Associated abnormalities of the vertebrae and upper urinary tract are common.

(c) Innervation of the pelvic musculature is often defective.

(d) The provision of adequate muscular control involves complicated and difficult surgical reconstruction by the sacro–abdomino–perineal approach.

Anorectal agenesis

This is the usual anomaly and is much more common in boys than in girls. In both sexes a fistula is almost always present.

121

In the common variety in boys there is a recto-urethral fistula. The clinical features are early obstruction, no opening in the perineum, and the passage of meconium in the urine. On straight x-ray the gas is at or above the 'M' point (*Figures 6.5a, 6.6a*).

Less commonly there is a rectovesical fistula. The clinical and radiological features are similar although obstruction may not be so severe. Straight x-rays may show air in the bladder (*Figure 6.7a*).

Very rarely there is no fistula and consequently complete obstruction with no meconium in the urine.

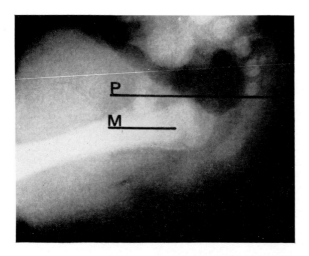

Figure 6.5a. Anorectal agenesis, inverted film showing gas-bubble level above 'M'

In all varieties the immediate treatment is colostomy and subsequent loopograms will confirm the site of termination of the bowel and show up the fistula when present (*Figures 6.5c, 6.6b, 6.7b, 6.7c*).

In the common variety in girls there is a fistula into the vault of the vagina (*Figure 6.8*). The clinical features are early obstruction, no opening in the perineum and the passage of meconium per vaginam. On separating the labia only two openings are visible, namely vagina and urethra, the fistula being out of sight. Straight x-rays may reveal a terminal gas shadow above the 'M' point if the obstruction is severe.

Less commonly the anatomy is more primitive and a urogenital sinus is present with a fistula into a cloacal canal (*Figure 6.9*).

122

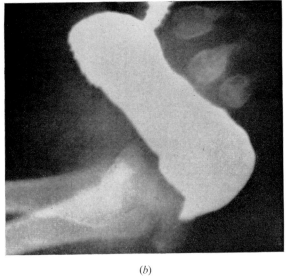

(b)

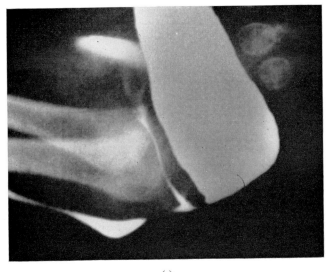

(c)

Figure 6.5b, c. Same case; loopogram showing anterior beaking of rectum and narrow fistula into the prostatic urethra

123

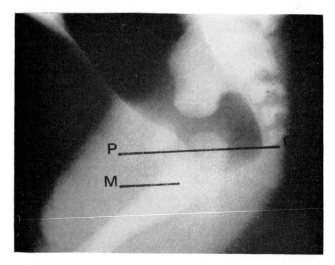

Figure 6.6a. Anorectal agenesis showing gas level above the 'M' point

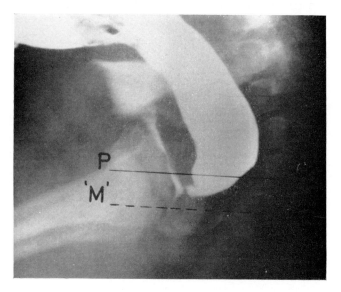

Figure 6.6b. Same case; loopogram showing fistula into prostatic urethra, note elongated bladder neck and typical posterior kinking of prostatic urethra at fistula site

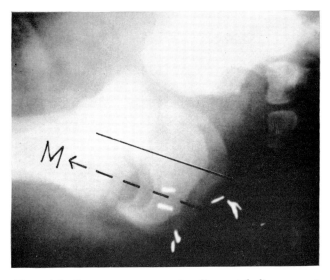

Figure 6.6c. Same case; post-operative film; metal clips were put along the pelvic insertion of the puborectalis and this film shows them in relation to ' M'

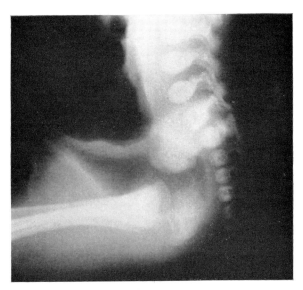

Figure 6.7a. Lateral film showing gas in the bladder from a rectovesical fistula

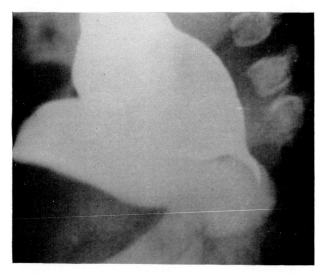

Figure 6.7b. Same case; loopogram showing the rectovesical fistula entering base of bladder and bladder filling from jet of contrast media

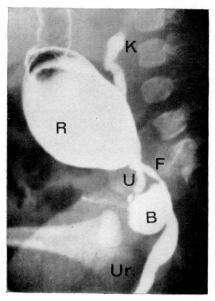

Figure 6.7c. Bladder (B) emptying into (Ur) urethra; (R) rectum filled from the loopogram; (F) fistula into back of bladder; reflux has occurred up (U) the ureter on one side and outlines (K) kidney pelvis

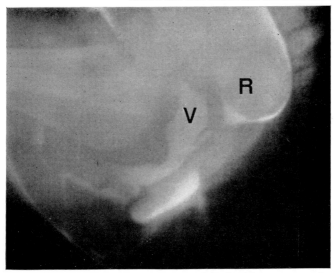

Figure 6.8. Loopogram showing rectovaginal fistula; (R) rectum contains a considerable amount of inspissated meconium

Figure 6.9. Cloacal abnormality; a Foley's catheter has been inserted up the (X) UG sinus and is seen in (B) bladder; some contrast has leaked back through a recto-cloacal fistula into (R) rectum and (C) colon

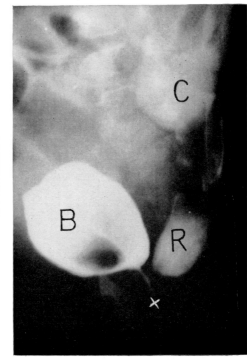

In all varieties the immediate treatment is colostomy and subsequent loopograms will outline the anatomy.

Rectal atresia

This very rare anomaly (2% of our cases) occurs in both boys

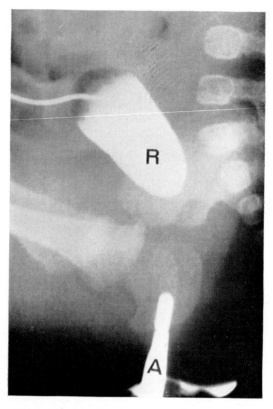

Figure 6.10. Rectal atresia: (R) rectum outlined by a loopogram from a short sigmoid colostomy; a thermometer has been inserted up the anal canal and reaches as far as the 'M' point. The perineum has been marked with barium paste

and girls. An anal canal is present but the rectum ends blindly above the pelvic floor. Obstructive symptoms develop early but the diagnosis may be missed because of the presence of an apparently normal anal canal. Straight x-rays show a terminal gas bubble well above the 'M' point and at a considerable distance from the tip of a thermometer inserted into the anus (*Figure 6.10*).

The immediate treatment is colostomy and subsequent loopograms will confirm the diagnosis and prove that no fistula is present.

INTERMEDIATE ANOMALIES

This group accounts for 15% of our cases. It includes a number of anomalies occurring in both boys and girls which, in the past, some

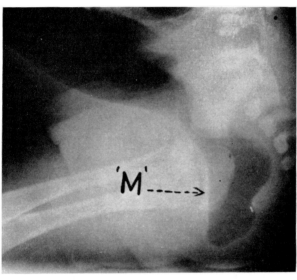

Figure 6.11. Anal agenesis; inverted film showing that gas has descended through the embracing puborectalis sling which posteriorly indents it at 'M'. This is an uncommon intermediate lesion which may give identical appearances to a completely low lesion

authorities have included with the high anomalies, while others have included them with the low anomalies. In their treatment the former workers have tended to use a sacro–abdomino–perineal approach for the reconstruction, while the latter have preferred a simple perineal anoplasty. We believe the initial treatment should be colostomy and have used an abdomino–perineal approach for the reconstruction at a later date.

Anal agenesis

Anal agenesis without fistula is rare (3%) in both boys and girls and the clinical presentation is similar to that of anorectal agenesis without fistula, an even rarer anomaly (see page 122). Straight x-rays will reveal the terminal gas shadow well below the 'M' point because only the distal anal canal is involved and the rectum is present and embraced by the puborectalis (*Figure 6.11*). The immediate treatment is colostomy and subsequent loopograms will confirm the diagnosis.

Anal agenesis with fistula is also rare in boys in whom the fistula opens into the bulbous part of the urethra (*Figure 6.12*). Clinically it presents exactly like anorectal agenesis with recto-urethral fistula,

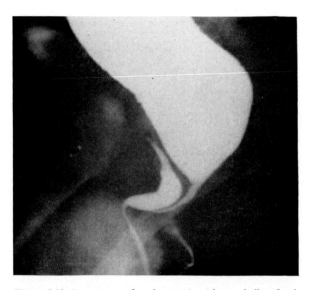

Figure 6.12. Loopogram of anal agenesis with rectobulbar fistula

i.e., early obstruction, no orifice in the perineum and the passage of meconium in the urine. Frequently an associated hypospadias is present. Provided obstruction exists the straight x-ray will reveal the terminal gas bubble below the 'M' point. The immediate treatment is colostomy and subsequent loopograms are necessary for accurate diagnosis.

In females the fistula may open low down in the vagina in which case it has to be differentiated from anorectal agenesis with fistula or low vestibular fistulae. This depends on visualizing the opening on colposcopy, but a fistulogram or subsequent loopogram is often necessary for accurate diagnosis (*Figure 6.13*). When a narrow fistula

130

opens into the vestibule the clinical presentation is similar to that of the various low anomalies with an opening at the vulvar site. However, a probe introduced into the orifice will pass cephalad and not dorsally. Fistulograms or subsequent loopograms are essential for accurate diagnosis.

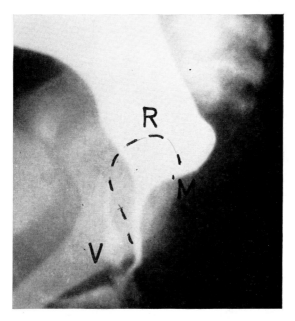

Figure 6.13. Anorectal agenesis with elongated fistula running down to the vestibule; (V) marks position of the vagina; the sacrum is partially absent

Anorectal stenosis

This is a rare lesion but important because it may be confused with anal stenosis. The stenosis involves the anus as well as the lower rectum and therefore abdominoperineal reconstruction is necessary. Fistulograms or subsequent loopograms are essential for diagnosis.

LOW OR TRANSLEVATOR ANOMALIES

These account for 40% of our cases. They occur in both boys and girls and are generally not serious anomalies. Obstruction is seldom severe and, if so, usually transient. Associated anomalies are not common, the pelvic nerves are intact and reconstruction usually involves only a simple perineal operation. However, unwarranted operations may have disastrous consequences.

In these babies the rectum is present and normal, but the anus is abnormal. The latter may be situated at the normal anal site, in the perineum anterior to the normal site, or in girls, in the vulva. An orifice is almost always present but it is usually stenosed.

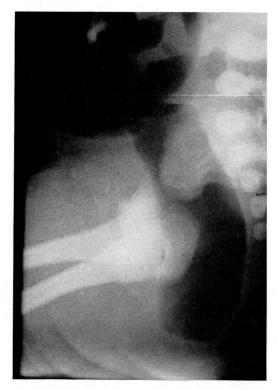

Figure 6.14a. Covered anus, gas has descended well down below the pelvic floor

At normal anal site

These anomalies are rare (5% of our cases) and include covered anus and anal stenosis, which is mostly a variant of covered anus (the pinhole anus of Denis Browne). Both types are more common in boys than in girls. In covered anus the meconium will be seen shining through the skin at the anal site and in anal stenosis the skin has ruptured leaving a tiny opening through which meconium exudes. Straight x-rays will reveal a terminal gas bubble below the 'M' point (*Figure 6.14a*). The diagnosis can be confirmed by injecting water soluble contrast into the bowel through the perineum (*Figure 6.14b*), but this is usually unnecessary.

At perineal site

Covered anus with anocutaneous fistula is very much more common in boys, in whom the diagnosis is self-evident; meconium can

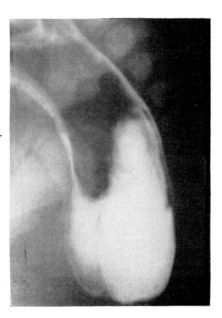

Figure 6.14b. Same case; rectum demonstrated by an injection of water soluble contrast media through the perineum; the meconium mass (negative filling defect) did not prevent the descent of gas in Figure 6.14a

be seen tracking beneath the skin in the midline from the site of the normal anus to the point of exit in the perineum or even further forward on to the raphe of the scrotum or the ventral surface of the penis. In girls the track of meconium is less easily identified but on passing a probe into the orifice in the perineum it passes directly backwards immediately subcutaneously. Further investigations are unnecessary but a fistulogram will confirm the diagnosis.

The anterior perineal anus is simply a slightly stenosed but

133

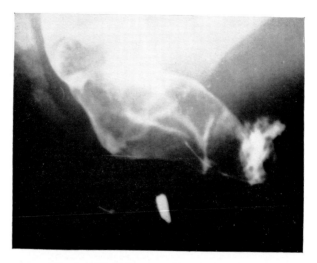

Figure 6.15. Vulvar anus shown by fistulogram

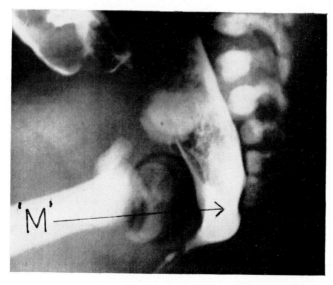

Figure 6.16. Fistulogram showing anovestibular fistula; the rectum has descended well down through the puborectalis sling which indents it posteriorly at 'M'; there is an air-filled balloon catheter in the vagina

normal anus placed forward of the normal site. In girls this gives the typical 'shot-gun perineum' appearance described by Denis Browne.

At vulvar site

An opening into the vulva close to the fourchette occurs in a number of low anomalies in girls.

The vulvar anus, also known as vestibular anus or vulvar ectopic anus, has the appearance of a normal anus (*Figure 6.15*).

The anovulvar fistula is a variant of covered anus and the opening has a ragged appearance.

In the anovestibular fistula the bowel has passed through the pubo-rectalis but an anal canal has not formed and the terminal bowel communicates with the vestibule through a small fistula (*Figure 6.16*).

In all three varieties a probe inserted into the orifice passes somewhat dorsally and not cephalad, as in the intermediate anomalies with fistulae; a fistulogram may be necessary for accurate diagnosis.

MISCELLANEOUS

These lesions, which include perineal grooves and complex lesions associated with extrophy of the bladder, are extremely uncommon and will not be discussed.

Bibliography and References

CHAPTER ONE
Bibliography
Holder, T. M. and Ashcraft, K. W. (1966). *Current Problems in Surgery.* Chicago; Year Book Medical Publishers.
Rickham, P. P. and Johnston, J. H. (1969). *Neonatal Surgery.* London; Butterworths. [Contains many useful references.]

References
Chrispin, A. R. (1969). 'Abnormalities of oesophageal function: some radiological aspects.' In *Recent Advances in Paediatric Surgery*, 2nd ed., Ed. by A. W. Wilkinson. London; Churchill.

CHAPTER TWO
Bibliography
Bell, R. S., Graham, C. B. and Stevenson, J. K. (1971). 'Roentgenologic and clinical manifestations of neonatal necrotising enterocolitis.' *Am. J. Roentgenol.*, **112**, 123.
Berdon, W. E. and Baker, D. H. (1972). *Pediatric X-ray Diagnosis*, 6th ed., Ed. by J. Caffey. Chicago; Year Book Medical Publishers.

CHAPTER THREE
Bibliography
Astley, R. (1956). *Radiology of the Alimentary Tract in Infancy.* London; Edward Arnold.
Singleton, E. D. (1959). *X-ray Diagnosis of the Alimentary Tract of Infants and Children.* Chicago; Year Book Medical Publishers.
[Both these books are good paediatric references, although they are a little dated concerning our neonatal problems.]

CHAPTER FOUR
Bibliography
Benson, C. D., Mustard, W. T., Ravitch, M. M., Snyder, W. H. and Welch, K. J. (1969). *Pediatric Surgery*, 2nd ed., Vol. II. Chicago; Year Book Medical Publishers.
Wagget, J., Bishop, H. C. and Koop, C. E. (1970). 'Experience with Gastrografin enema in the treatment of meconium ileus.' *J. pediat. Surg.*, **5**, 649.

CHAPTER FIVE

Bibliography

Bell, R. S., Graham, C. B. and Stevenson, J. K. (1971). 'Roentgenologic and clinical manifestations of neonatal necrotising enterocolitis.' *Am. J. Roentgenol.*, **112**, 123.

Berdon, W. E. and Baker, D. H. (1972). *Pediatric X-ray Diagnosis*, 6th ed., Ed. by J. Caffey. Chicago; Year Book Medical Publishers.

Ehrenpreis, T. (1970). *Hirschsprung's Disease*. Chicago; Year Book Medical Publishers. [This book *gives a complete bibliography of references quoted and* is essential reading for further study in Hirschsprung's disease.]

Hope, J. W., Borns, P. F. and Berg, P. K. (1965). 'Roentgenological manifestations of Hirschsprung's disease in infancy.' *Am. J. Roentgenol.*, **95**, 217.

References

Ehrenpreis, T. and Pernow, B. (1952). 'On the occurrence of substance P in the rectosigmoid in Hirschsprung's disease.' *Acta physiol. scand.*, **27**, 380.

— Norberg, K. A. and Wirsen, C. (1968). 'Sympathetic innervation of the colon in Hirschsprung's disease: a histochemical study.' *J. pediat. Surg.*, **3**, 43.

Kamijo, K., Hiatt, R. B. and Koelle, G. B. (1953). 'Congenital megacolon: a comparison of the spastic and hypertrophied segments with respect to cholinesterase activities and sensitivities to acetylcholine, DFP and the barium ion.' *Gastroenterology*, **24**, 173.

Lawson, J. O. N. and Nixon, H. H. (1967). 'Anal canal pressures in the diagnosis of Hirschsprung's disease.' *J. pediat. Surg.*, **2**, 544.

MacMahon, R. A., Cohen, S. J. and Eckstein, H. B. (1963). 'Colostomies in infancy and childhood.' *Archs dis. Child.*, **38**, 114.

Okomoto, E. and Ueda, T. (1967). 'Embryogenesis of intramural ganglia of the gut and its relation to Hirschsprung's disease.' *J. pediat. Surg.*, **2**, 437.

Swenson, O. and Fisher, J. H. (1959). 'Hirschsprung's disease in the newborn.' *Archs. Surg.*, **97**, 734.

Tobon, F., Reid, N. C. R. W., Talbert, J. L. and Schuster, M. M. (1968). 'Non-surgical test for the diagnosis of Hirschsprung's disease.' *N. Engl. J. Med.*, **278**, 188.

Wright, P. G. and Sheppard, J. J. (1965). 'Response to drugs of isolated human colonic muscle.' *Lancet*, **2**, 1161.

Yntema, C. C. and Hammond, W. S. (1954). 'Origin of intrinsic ganglia of trunk viscera from vagal neural crest in chick embryo.' *J. comp. Neurol.*, **101**, 515.

CHAPTER SIX
Bibliography
Stephens, F. D. and Smith, E. D. (1971). *Anorectal Malformations in Children*. Chicago; Year Book Medical Publishers.
Cremin, B. J. (1971). 'The radiological assessment of anorectal anomalies.' *Radiology*, **22**, 239.
Louw, J. H. (1965). *Current Problems in Surgery*. Chicago; Year Book Medical Publishers.

Index

141

INDEX